WHAT WOULD VIRGINIA WOOLF DO?

WHAT WOULD VIRGINIA WOOLF DO?

**And Other Questions
I Ask Myself as I Attempt to
Age Without Apology**

NINA LOREZ COLLINS

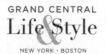

GRAND CENTRAL
Life & Style
NEW YORK · BOSTON

(Cover and interior design by Eight and a Half, New York, Ltd.
Design: Bonnie Siegler and Kristen Ren * Painting: Jeff Scher)

Grand Central Life & Style
Hachette Book Group
1290 Avenue of the Americas, New York, NY 10104
grandcentrallifeandstyle.com
twitter.com/grandcentralpub

First Edition: April 2018

Grand Central Life & Style is an imprint of Grand Central Publishing. The Grand Central Life & Style name and logo are trademarks of Hachette Book Group, Inc.

The publisher is not responsible for websites (or their content) that are not owned by the publisher.

The Hachette Speakers Bureau provides a wide range of authors for speaking events. To find out more, go to www.hachettespeakersbureau.com or call (866) 376-6591.

Library of Congress Cataloging-in-Publication Data has been applied for.

ISBNs: 978-1-5387-2795-9 (hardcover), 978-1-5387-2796-6 (ebook)

Printed in the United States of America

LSC-C

10 9 8 7 6 5 4 3 2 1

TO MARGARET LEE,

WHO CONCEIVED OUR HILARIOUS NAME
AND HAS BEEN THE WITTY AND SAGE
GODMOTHER OF THE GROUP SINCE DAY ONE

CONTENTS

CHAPTER FOUR: PAGE 122

(PARENTING)

A (Not Quite) Empty Nest

Has It Been Eighteen Years Already? * Big Kids, Big Problems * The Happiness Paradox * Coping with Aging While Bending Over to Pick up the Lego Bricks * Before I Forget…the Bright Side * It's Official: French Women Are Better at Everything * Grab Your Baggage, We're Going on a Guilt Trip * A Note on Our Own Miserable Childhoods * Have You Seen My Boundaries? * Weaning Kids from the Financial Tit * First Departures * The Ten Best Things About the Empty Nest * The Ten Worst Things About the Empty Nest * They're Back…

CHAPTER FIVE: PAGE 156

(BEAUTY)

Mirror, Mirror…?

Are My Botox Treatments Contributing to the "New Normal"? * Fraxel, Juvéderm, Peels…Pick Your Poison * The Deepest Cut: Plastic Surgery * Long in the Tooth * Crepey Neck Skin? * Not by the Hair on My Chinny Chin Chin * Beyond the Tweezer * Eyelash Extensions—Yes, Eyelash Extensions * Fifty Shades of Gray Hair * Hair Loss * Pubic Knowledge: Waxing, Dying… Transplants?! * OPPP—Other People's Products and Philosophies * The High Cost of Beauty * I'm Okay, You're Okay: Acceptance and Solidarity

CHAPTER SIX: PAGE 195

(EMOTIONS)

Anxiety and Depression and Stress, Oh My!

I Am Woman, Hear Me Whimper * Not Waving, or Drowning, or Even Sleeping * Why Are We So Depressed? * So What to Do About It? Prozac (and Xanax and Valium) Nation * How Bad Do I Have It? * Am I Really

CONTENTS

WHAT WOULD VIRGINIA WOOLF DO?

(A NOTE ABOUT THE TITLE)

IT'S MEANT TO BE IRONIC. If you are a Virginia Woolf scholar, you may well still enjoy this book, but please don't take me to task for using her name in vain. I'm a reasonably well-read feminist and a fan. I loved *A Room of One's Own* when I read it in college, and I once wrote a twenty-page graduate school paper on *To the Lighthouse*. *Moments of Being*, a collection of Woolf's autobiographical writings, is my favorite book of hers, and I'm interested in the whole Bloomsbury history. But the title of this book came about because Woolf is a kick-ass woman of letters who killed herself in her fifties. As I was starting perimenopause and dealing with myriad symptoms that were bringing me down, "What Would Virginia Woolf Do?" struck me as a very funny line. It still does.

AND ANOTHER THING

Some names of Woolfers and other friends have been changed to protect privacy and others have not. All stories are true and any mistakes are mine and mine alone.

INTRODUCTION

AGING,
IT'S (NOT) FOR PUSSIES

You need a cohort of peers to go through the aging process with you.
A cackle of crones! A cavalry!
—MARINA BENJAMIN, *THE MIDDLEPAUSE: ON TURNING FIFTY*

IN THE FALL OF THE YEAR I turned forty-six, I started experiencing night sweats and hot flashes. My periods had been erratic over the course of the previous year, so after a few weeks of worried confusion, I began to wonder if the symptoms might be the onset of perimenopause, the phase in a woman's life I understood to precede menopause, but about which I knew little. A week or two later, I was waking up every night between three and five a.m. As someone who has been a lifelong excellent sleeper, this turn of events was deeply disconcerting. Naturally, I went straight to Google.

Efficiently directed to Healthline.com, I found sleeplessness among the many symptoms of perimenopause. On top of the sleep troubles, hot flashes, and night sweats, the site lists an alarming thirty-three additional symptoms, including feelings of dread, apprehension, and doom. Other winners are head and/or pubic hair loss, increase in facial hair, gastrointestinal distress, indigestion, flatulence, itchy skin, and nausea. The list goes on and on, each ailment more depressing than the next: mood swings, depression, thinning nails, anxiety, changes in body odor, lack of libido. Upon further investigation, I learned that the median length of time women endure symptoms is 7.4 years, and typically longer, if you are like me and the symptoms start before menstruation ceases. It appears likely, from what I've read, that I'll be going through this "change of life" for about eleven years. That's a long time to go from youngish to oldish, which, if we're going to be brutally frank, is essentially what this phase is all about.

I had my kids early. I delivered my first child at twenty-four and my last at thirty. In New York City, where I live, this is fairly unusual. Because as women we make so many of our long-lasting friendships through our children, one thing it means is that practically all of my girlfriends are older than me, generally by a decade, so somewhere between fifty and sixty at this point. They had already gone through this! As I found myself sweaty, exhausted, and depressed in the fall of 2015, I was surprised that not a single one had warned me. Wasn't the emergence of back fat alone worth a conversation?

I soon realized the reason women don't talk openly about aging is pretty straightforward. We've been raised in a world, indoctrinated into a whole value system, in which young equals good and old equals bad, and we're embarrassed to admit that we're crossing that line. Who wants to sit around moaning about hormonal decline? It makes us feel pathetic. Even worse, it makes us question our intrinsic worth. Of course, some lucky women don't experience menopausal or perimenopausal symptoms so dramatically. Some don't have any symptoms at all. But even those women, like all of the rest of us, deal with the larger issues. Namely, what does it mean and feel like to be "older" in an ageist society—especially for females?

Any attempt to engage my children or husband in a conversation about my sleeplessness and other premenopausal woes was met with glazed-over stares of incomprehension and flat-out disinterest. No one wants to hear this stuff over the dinner table, and if you're not in it, you truly cannot, and do not, want to relate. Yet I felt an urgent need to talk.

So I created a group on Facebook and called it "What Would Virginia Woolf Do?" The official description of the group is: "A closed, confidential forum for women over forty, with a bent toward the literary, witty, and feminist. A place to discuss, support, and share things we may not care to share with the men and children in our lives." From the start, the group grew exponentially from friends to friends of friends to strangers, everyone wanting to know they weren't alone—or going crazy.

Going on three years later, what has emerged (exploded, actually— we're up to just under eight thousand members and growing) is a surprisingly candid, lively, and intimate extended conversation representing the range of interests of women in our cohort: educated, sophisticated, savvy, literary, and politically minded women who have strong opinions and a fierce sense of humor. We come from all over the country, even the world, and we talk about feminism, our bodies, health, fashion, politics, culture, men, and of course sex.

Everything is up for grabs, but interestingly, we're less preoccupied with our children than with ourselves. And I've noticed that we're not that obsessed with our careers either. This is a time in life when we want to think about *meaning*, about purpose, about how to be our best selves and how to love ourselves as we enter the second half of our lives. We yearn to acknowledge the nostalgia and sadness that come with age, but we also want to revel in our hard-earned wisdom. Women really do want to talk about these things, desperately, but they need a safe forum in which to do it.

According to the last US census, there are nearly 126 million adult women in the United States, more than 40 million of whom are ages forty to sixty. More than anything, the experience of these conversations made me acutely aware of a broader reality. There are literally millions of Gen X women yearning for the kind of support and information that will help us age gracefully, but without pandering or dumbing down—or making us nod off earlier than we already do. We want a resource that's filled with humor, intelligence, and sexiness along with practical, rigorously researched information, and serving that need can't be fully realized by a Facebook group. I wanted to dive deeper into the issues and write on a larger canvas about the profound and sometimes difficult journey we are making.

So much cultural attention is paid to girls' coming-of-age, but very little to this other moment when women enter a significant new stage in life. There's clearly room for a broader conversation around what it all means, how it feels, and the best way to navigate this new territory. The aim of this book is to provide a manifesto for the next coming-of-age. We need to be able to share our darkest stuff and know that we will be heard. (What does it feel like when your man needs Viagra for the first time? What's it like to be envious of your college-age daughter? Am I drinking too much? Can I just say that sometimes I hate the way my body is changing?) How can we experience this change feeling empowered, not diminished?

Full disclosure: in many ways for me this whole project has been about debunking shame, or at the very least providing a forum where we can go from isolated shame to shared solutions. As women we're told way too often that there's something wrong with us, and there isn't. Nothing you or I have experienced—in our bodies, our homes, our relationships—is new, but what is novel is that we have the opportunity to talk about it all out in the open, and that actually might help us feel better. So I don't hold back. There may be times when you don't agree with what I do or say, and you might not always like me, but that's okay, because none of us is likable all the time and we're all still worthy of love.

For the record, I'm divorced and a mother of four. I'm also mixed race (half-black and half-white) and straight, and although I was raised by poor artists, I'm now what would be considered by some Trumpians as a "liberal elite." I live in Brooklyn, for Christ's sake. So if the sensibility of the book skews in any of those directions, you now know why and I hope you aren't offended.

Virginia Woolf was a contradiction. She killed herself in her fifties, and yet in many ways she represents all that we aspire to: a brilliant feminist, a wit, a woman of guts and glamour. Woolf's famous "room of one's own" is what women still need, and what we crave more than ever as we enter this new phase of life. This book provides resources, but much more: I hope it's an intimate destination that showcases what happens when women feel comfortable enough to get real with each other.

What you have here in your hands is not just a book about peri-menopause or menopause—you might not even be there yet—but a companion, a funny and insightful girlfriend to accompany you on the road after forty. I don't want a ten-pound tome that screams "menopause" on my nightstand, but I do want frank and intimate conversation mixed with anecdotes and honesty. If it's wrapped up in a literary joke, all the better. A place that makes me feel sexy, real, challenged, and informed all at the same time? A place to seek solace and laugh at the stuff no one seems to be talking about in public (yet)? That's a place I want to be, and I want to be there with you.

Some people go to priests; others to poetry; I to my friends.

—VIRGINIA WOOLF

WARNING LABELS

Who are we? I'll let the women speak for themselves. Here's an early post to the group, and a sampling of unattributed answers.

If you were forced to wear a Warning Label, what would yours say?

Does not suffer fools gladly

Unapologetic feminist

Sunny with a chance of showers

May cause laughter

Scary when hungry

Bored easily

Don't tread on me

Not all original parts

Flammable when pissed

Though she be but little, she is fierce

Long-lasting when responsibly nurtured

Occasionally says fuck

Handle with care. Combustible.

Handle with care. Fragile.

Way tougher than I look

Lie to me at your peril

I bite!

If I'm crying, I'm frustrated...not sad.

Nasty woman comin' at ya!

Likely gonna hug you

Smart, and I know it

Slippery when wet

If this van is a rockin', don't come a knockin'

Fork in the road ahead

Gets better with age

Helpless to control sarcasm

Easy weeper

Iron fist in a velvet glove

Irrationally happy

Unrepentant bitch

Overwhelmed introvert

Short fuse

I just want peace

No small talk

I'm guessing you already feel among friends, so let's keep going...

CHAPTER ONE

(FASHION)

DEATH BY EILEEN FISHER AND OTHER FASHION TRAGEDIES

Vain trifles as they seem, clothes have, they say,
more important offices than to merely keep us warm.
They change our view of the world and the world's view of us.
—VIRGINIA WOOLF

IT'S FIVE P.M. ON A Tuesday back when I still had kids at home and I'm returning from Fairway supermarket in my pajamas. My tennis elbow (a repetitive stress injury sustained not from racket sports but likely from too many hand jobs) is killing me and has not been helped by heaving jumbo-sized containers of laundry detergent into a grocery cart. I text my seventeen-year-old daughter and ask her to come help me with the groceries (it's the only way I know I can reliably reach her, except maybe by Snapchat, whatever that is). She says she's busy but will come down in a bit, and I'm too tired to argue, so I wait. I sit in my Subaru Outback, parked in the lot behind our building, and dip into the latest tome on menopause that has arrived from Amazon. These sorts of books have comprised my reading list for the last few months, as they have for tens of thousands of other women searching for peace of mind and advice.

Twenty minutes later, after I've finished a chapter on the cheery subject of uterine prolapse, my beloved child shows up, looking both sexy and adorable in a denim miniskirt, skimpy tank top, and my old Yves Saint Laurent black suede thigh-high boots. At five-four and 115 pounds, with long, blond, curly hair, perfect C cups, and many piercings, she basically looks like a twenty-first-century version of Daisy Duke (and because you're my age, you'll get that reference). Before she can get to me, a group of random men snapping pictures of a Lamborghini in the adjacent park intercept her to ask if she'll pose by the car for them. True story. Again: I'm in my pajamas, with a station wagon full of groceries and an aching arm. And a couple of pimples on the lower right side of my face. I don't feel jealous, just weary.

A reasonable question to ask is, "Why is she wearing her pajamas at five p.m. on a Tuesday afternoon?" There are a few answers to that question: I was having a brutal week of what I could only hope was PMS—I hadn't had my period in two months, my breasts were sore, and I had seemingly put on ten pounds overnight, was having headaches, and was so tired I could barely get through the day. That afternoon I had called it quits early and at two p.m. took a bath, slipped into my pj's (which generally consist of some sort of quasi-sexy lingerie-like top and Bedhead bottoms), and crawled into bed for a nap. With my vibrator.

An hour later I remembered that we didn't have milk, eggs, or bread—or a plan for dinner. My last child (of four) is around for only a few more months, and on the rare evenings she and my second husband and I are all going to be together at home, I still (sometimes) valiantly try to make an effort. So I threw on a sweater and headed out to the grocery store.

The other part of the answer is that pajamas are comfortable, and they are easy to wear, and sometimes I don't give a shit anymore about what anybody else thinks—I'll wear what I damn well please. And if I'm being honest, I generally assume no one's really looking anyway. This is also a tendency I must have inherited from my own mother, whom I fondly recall driving me to school in her flannel nightgowns, high ruffled collar and all. Mortified at the time, I remember begging her to drop me off a block away from the building, but now I really get it. And so do the multitudes of other women my age who wear sweats and jammies in public without thinking twice.

My teenage girl, of course, is experiencing the flip side of being almost invisible: being gawked at and objectified, with an amateur photography fan club on practically every corner. She probably put on her outfit hoping to look cute, especially to her friends, and wasn't thinking about the fact that complete strangers might have a stake in her fashion choices. While on the outside all that attention is an ego booster, on the inside, it's also oppressive. Walking around in your pajamas in broad daylight can be an act of liberation.

This got me to thinking about fashion in midlife in general. I do have to actually get dressed most days, and it's often hard to figure out what to wear. Every time I leave the house I feel more pressure to consider, "Can I actually pull this off?" and it's stressful and depressing to feel this crisis of confidence. I feel like I should be well beyond these sorts of feelings at this stage of my life.

The crux of the problem is multifold: on the one hand, I don't want to be relegated to certain "older lady" norms or to feel like my options are shrinking. That's just adding insult to injury, for Christ's sake, what with hot flashes and vaginal atrophy. But on the other hand, a lot of what I already own—jeans, cute dresses, tight skirts—makes me feel like I'm trying too hard. For example, at some point, I just decided that shorts looked "bad" on me. What does that even mean? Will the sight of my less-than-taut and slightly crepey legs burn somebody's eyeballs out? What standards do I feel the need to conform to?

As I start to slide toward the older side of the aging spectrum, I suddenly worry much more about whether I look "appropriate," but even more important, whether what I'm wearing still makes me feel like "me," like the person I still think of myself as. The truth is that I, like probably all of us, have internalized some sort of negative value that society tells me I have over a certain age, when I'm no longer "ripe," with perky breasts and lustrous skin and hair. That's beyond screwy, and it translates to a sort of immobility, a feeling of being frozen when I stand in my closet and consider my options.

A 2013 consumer studies report by Goldman Sachs points out that women's spending on clothes peaks at forty-four, then "goes into a long slump." For some women, middle age marks a point when we honestly aren't as concerned with fashion and style as we used to be, but it's much more complicated than that. Not only are our bodies changing in ways that aren't accommodated by the latest trends, but the message is loud and clear that after a certain point, we should dispense with all sorts of items, from shorter skirts to sleeveless blouses. The rules, of course, are arbitrary, but still, many of us have swallowed them. Most women's fashion magazines publish a splashy annual "Age" issue, purportedly to celebrate women of every generation. What the substance boils down to is a decade-by-decade breakdown of what you should and should not wear in your twenties, thirties, forties, fifties, and occasionally sixties (above which age, presumably, you are truly irrelevant to the fashion industry). So, according to this logic, what if you donned, say, a leather motorcycle jacket that's deemed cool for a twenty-nine-year-old when you are forty-one—will you spontaneously combust?

What choices are we left with exactly? Anything that's considered more "age appropriate"—looser clothes, suits, "slacks" (ew), even yoga or exercise clothes—makes me feel so old and fading that I can't stand it. Fashion in midlife bounces off an inherent paradox: our bodies are starting to feel unruly, like they are betraying us (chin hair, paunch, skin sag), and at the same time there are suddenly both more rules *and* fewer choices.

To my mind, the solution to this quandary is a combination of humor and defiance with a healthy dollop of self-awareness. As a good friend said recently, "I wear mom jeans, Crocs, bathing suits with skirts, and could give a crap what anyone thinks." Rock on, sister. As the designer Anne Klein said, "Clothes aren't going to change the world. The women who wear them will."

The bright side is that this phase of life really can be a great opportunity for reinvention. Figuring out what I want to look like, and how I want to feel in what I'm wearing, is what it's all about. It's not an easy process. Some of us may revel in the relief of saying goodbye to tube tops and others may mourn letting go of an item that is a poignant reminder of their younger selves. But let's face it: as long as we're not wearing a hospital gown or a colostomy bag, it's all good, just best done with some ownership and thought. For me personally—and this may change—that means wearing high clogs and clothes that veer toward pajamas and lingerie.

THE TYRANNY OF HEELS—AND WHY I LOVE THEM

Sensuality doesn't come from heels—
especially if you can't walk in them.
It's like a beautiful woman who has
the perfect hair and makeup but doesn't smile.
You should dress to feel good, not show off.
It takes life to learn that.
—INÈS DE LA FRESSANGE

PART OF WHAT'S SO APPEALING about clogs is that I'm less and less able to wear high heels, which makes me want to cry. I was never a Carrie Bradshaw–like stiletto wearer. Even in my ultrayouth, my feet were wide and stilettos made me feel like an unsteady giraffe. But I remember wearing four-high-inch pumps to high school (driving there in my $250 yellow VW Bug with the rusted-out floor), and my entire adult life I've worn towering wedges and chunky high-heeled boots—shoes that practically feel like signature items. I love everything about heels: how they enhance my legs (one of my better features), how tall I become (my real height is a solid but not impressive five foot six), and how sexy and powerful they make me feel.

However, as great as heels are, being able to walk upright on two feet is even better. It's been a slow process, but around three years ago I started feeling ever so slightly unsafe that far off the ground. It dawned on me that I could easily twist or even break an ankle. I said good-bye to five inches forever. Maybe it was the recognition of my own mortality, starting from the feet up. Since then, I have in fact teetered a few times, and I even tripped and fell on a sidewalk once last Christmas Eve after too much to drink. More and more I find myself gripping my husband's arm as we hurry somewhere. I do yoga, and my balance is respectable (tree position is not a problem, even with my arms straight up above my head!), but the fact is that I'm just plain getting older and my center of gravity is unfortunately shifting upward toward my waist and midriff. The writing is on the wall. I can see that in a few years I'll be going down to three inches, then two, and then flats... This is why, clogs.

I'm not nearly alone here. We're giving up heels either for safety or, even more commonly, because it hurts too goddamn much to wear them now. According to the Illinois Podiatric Medical Association, women are four times more likely than men to have foot problems, generally a consequence of high heels. For one thing, pregnancy hormones weaken feet, and women are at a higher risk of stress fractures in the foot than men. Also, more than half of women get bunions, and women are nine times as likely as men to have the problem, according to the American Academy of Orthopaedic Surgeons. Some doctors say the growing popularity of high heels and pointy-toed shoes, including among very young women, has helped increase the incidence of bunions. In any case, I'm sure it hasn't been lost on you that foot surgery for women in their fifties appears to be epidemic. In the last two years, I've had six friends undergo operations that sound utterly barbaric. Whether it's damage and calcification sustained from years of pinched high heels, too much running on concrete, or simply life and genetics, they have all had procedures that involved slicing and shaving bones, inserting pins, and weeks and weeks of bed rest and crutches. And you only have one foot done at a time! After a year or so of full recovery, you can look forward to going through it all over again with the other foot! This is cruel and unusual, even by most standards of beauty sacrifice. Do men have these surgeries? Rarely. Why would they? They wear comfortable, supportive flat shoes all their lives. They don't contort themselves into death-defying contraptions to look sexy and winsome. When you think about it, the whole thing is devastatingly messed up.

Writer Mary Karr bemoaned this ugly reality in a 2016 article for *The New Yorker*. At age sixty, she described her once-perfect feet as gnarled, beleaguered, and bunioned. She taped up a box of high heels that might have funded an early retirement and sent them off to Goodwill. She notes Michelle Obama's (sensible) love of kitten heels as well as Victoria Beckham's recent announcement that even her days of high heels are over. Following in Karr's pained footsteps, Cindi Leive, editor in chief of *Glamour*, chronicled her own experiment with wearing flats for a week straight. Emotionally, it was hard—she hated feeling short, and consequently less commanding, but boy was it comfortable. Grieving over having to chuck all of our prettiest shoes is a real thing, an issue of identity for many of us, and as I type this I gaze longingly at the pile of high heels in my closet. I feel sad for the day when they'll all be replaced by shoes that are far more practical but much less attractive.

My dear friend Kamy, a youthful forty-three, recently developed plantar fasciitis, seemingly out of nowhere (kind of like my elbow, natch). Her doctor told her she had to start wearing these ugly orthopedic inserts, stat, and she ignored him, because she can't wear inserts with flip-flops, or Manolos, or pretty much anything but sneakers. A month later she was back in his office, practically crying in pain. He reiterated, in no uncertain terms, that she needed to wear the inserts, and then gave her a brochure full of the ugliest bejeweled old-lady shoes known to womankind. He said, "You can wear any of these." That was when she started to cry for real.

Hopefully, your predicament isn't as bad as poor Kamy's. If you aren't being commanded to wear orthopedic inserts, and you haven't had recent foot surgery, you may just need, like me, to start considering other looks. I simply cannot wear four-inch anything (even clogs) much longer.

What are the options? Woolfers recommend Birkenstocks over pretty much everything else; also Clarks and Fit Flops! But you don't have to go straight from vertiginous pumps to earth shoes. Thankfully, there are designers making kitten heels, ballet flats (I hear Repetto are great), stylish sandals, low wedges, et cetera. Did all those shoe companies suddenly realize that legions of women with aching feet also possess credit cards? It's about time. Even Christian Louboutin, who once said, "To feel like a woman, wear heels, to feel like a goddess, wear five inches," has been quietly producing lots of glam, low-heeled styles (glitter, patent leather, spikes, satin). For another fancy option, my friend Ann swears by the lower heeled Valentino Rockstud pumps. There are groovy sneakers from Converse to Lanvin, which can be worn with any number of outfits (skirts, jeans, dresses; I'm a firm believer that cute sneaks work with almost anything—I love to wear them with dresses). And funky sneakers are such a practical option for women who race from work to school to errands to volunteer work and sometimes feel like we are running from, not with, the wolves! Low-heeled boots also come in all sorts of awesome styles, and wearing a solid kick-ass boot can give you the mojo of a high heel—without the agony.

CLOGS: GIVING UP OR A SEXY SOLUTION TO SORE FEET?

I'VE BEEN WEARING VERSIONS OF CLOGS since around the seventh grade. (I think Dr. Scholl's count, right?) What's not to like? Comfortable, easy to slip on and off (great for airport security!), and they come in a million colors, styles, heights, and range of prices. Clogs have made a big comeback in the last few years and, unlike many footwear crazes, have had remarkable staying power. Part of the appeal might be nostalgic. We wore them as girls—one friend has sweet memories of shopping with her dad for an annual pair of red clogs, beginning in kindergarten—as did our role models. Writing for *New York* magazine about the trend, Allison P. Davis reminisced, "My style has long been inspired by my zany…art teacher…lots of eccentric dresses, 'artfully' unkempt hair, and, of course…the preferred sensible shoe: the clog."

They can be damn sexy too. Clogs are leg lengthening and feminine (which is why they look funny on men, at least to me), and even with the clomping, they still give the allure of a heel without the precarious balance and pinched toes. I bought my favorite pair ever, a high-end, four-inch, black Prada version with silver studs where the leather meets the wood, about eight years ago at a consignment shop. Walking the dog in these shoes, as old and scuffed up as they are, makes me feel like I'm in Paris, or like I could pick up the next man who crosses my path. Even at seven a.m.

For the winter I have a pair of black No.6 clog boots with shearling that peeps out at the ankle. They're not delicate in the least, but something about the design makes them perfect with almost anything—jeans, skirts, even certain dresses, all while enabling me to stay warm, walk in snow, do whatever the day calls for. And like my summer pair, they look hot.

REQUIEM FOR A THONG (PANTIES, NOT SHOES!)

AS MUCH AS I LOVE HEELS, I hate thongs. Always have. I prefer to go commando (and often do) rather than wear a piece of thread up my ass. And they only seem scarier to me as I age. God bless you if you love them, but the sight of my own cellulite-puckered, floppy ass in a thong is enough to send me to bed with the curtains closed for the rest of the day. I actually consider myself very lucky to have grown up before thongs and thickly padded push-up bras became de rigueur in the early aughts. I suspect it's no coincidence that the first network broadcast of the Victoria's Secret Fashion Show aired in 2001. As a young woman, I think I may have been sent over the edge by some of the underwear pressure my daughters see as commonplace. Wear whichever panties and bra make you feel comfortable, of course, but my opinion is, free the nip and cover the crack!

Fact: grandmothers actually wear granny panties, and I have the pictures to prove it. For years, my grandmother wore the exact same lingerie. Plunging high-waisted negligees that showed off her beautiful cleavage and sensible but pretty lace bra and panty sets. And one day, it was all gone, replaced by industrial bras that looked like they were produced behind the Iron Curtain in 1952 and huge cotton underwear in white or pale pink. "What gives?" I wondered.

I'm not quite there, but I do relate. I still love gorgeous bras and panties in fun colors (I love the look of a fuchsia bra strap, for example, peeking out from a simple black or white T-shirt), but my favorite panties are increasingly the über-simple cotton Hanky Panky bikinis in size large. (And I'm a basic size six in clothing; what decent-looking options does that leave for curvier women?) I like full ass coverage with lace trim. And cotton so my vagina can breathe, of course! Anything smaller feels to me like I'm accentuating my stomach and hip bulge. And anything larger, like a hipster or boy short, visually chops my midsection and thighs, about which I'm already self-conscious. I've become the Goldilocks of underwear. Too small, too big, too shiny, too boring. Out of fear that the exact style of my precious panties will be discontinued, I've stockpiled enough pairs to last through a nuclear winter.

Bras these days are a moving target. I'm droopier and also bigger, and the combination can make me feel a little sad sometimes. There are moments, after a shower, when I look at myself in the bathroom mirror and see the body of my aging aunt Francine. It used to be easy to feel sexy in any new black bra, and that's gotten harder. Maybe it's the recently acquired layer of back fat. (What's the evolutionary reason for this? Am I supposed to hibernate for the winter?) Or could it be the general, ever-so-slight tree-trunk thing that is happening with my torso? There's also the underarm pooch spilling over the edges of the underwire cups, which probably doesn't help. All these factors conspire to make finding the right bra a new challenge and make me wish things were different.

We all do that at times in our lives, right? Did you ever pray to a fairy godmother that you'd have way bigger breasts? Or much smaller ones? Well, she was very busy and waited until you were super-comfortable with your whatever-sized boobs to grant you that particular wish. Like my grandmother, I wore the same bra size since essentially the time I purchased my first bra, and then one morning I woke up with a significantly larger bustline. The experience can be surreal. I remember it clearly because it happened on a family vacation in a hotel room in California and my daughter opened her eyes and laughed out loud. The experience was not unlike when my milk came in for my first baby and, all of a sudden, I viscerally understood the expression "torpedo tits." While my husband is enchanted with this unexpected boon (given that my ass seems to have developed a slow leak, it's lucky that he's made the transition to "breast man"), buying a whole new bra—and underwear and nightgown—wardrobe is exasperating and expensive, but sometimes unavoidable if you want to keep your dignity.

Part of what makes finding clothes—and the stuff that goes under the clothes—that fit well and feel good is the inevitable shape-shifting that comes with aging. As we wend our way through these middle years, we seemingly, from one moment to the next, lose control of the one thing that's truly ours, our bodies. Alejandra Belmar, owner of the Brooklyn exercise franchise Everyday Athlete, says, "No amount of exercise will 'spot tone' batwings or a post-pregnancy paunch, nor will dieting restore one's hip to waist ratio to the ideal that clothing manufacturers design for." If you've developed a fondness for drawstrings and elastic waistbands, you are not alone, my friend. Some of the physical changes are unexpected and weird—you pull out a favorite dress from last summer and this year it's unbearably tight in a bizarre spot, like your shoulders or, often, your breasts.

In addition to basic weight gain (the average American woman puts on a pound a year from age forty to age sixty), lower hormone levels can increase the amount of fatty tissue in women's breasts and decrease the strength of the connective tissue (read: larger, saggier boobs). Or they shrink! It's a roll of the genetic dice. What's helpful for me is going to a professional bra store staffed with older, wiser women who are nonjudgmental, who really know their stuff, and who can fit you like the experts they are. Danny Koch, the fourth-generation owner of the Town Shop, an eighty-year-old Manhattan institution famous for its individualized fittings, puts it this way: "A seven-year-old bra is not going to do you any favors—the underwire is bent, the elastic stretched out. Gravity has a bad effect on people. What we are doing with a well-fitted bra is keeping your breasts as close to your chin as possible—for as long as possible. Just like with the ligaments in your knees, once they are stretched out, they aren't going to bounce back." Forget your high school 34Bs. Show your girls some love, whatever their size may be, with a comfortable, properly proportioned new bra.

TO SPANX OR NOT TO SPANX

A FEW YEARS AGO MY FRIEND "B" went to the annual gala for the Moth in New York City. All dressed up and underlayered with Spanx to hold it all in and accentuate her curves in the right places, at three a.m. she found herself in a dark bar making out with a well-known celebrity, an actor I'll describe as our age and sexy as hell in a slightly grungy sort of way. He started feeling her up, and she was totally into it—but every time his hand started inching up her bare leg under her dress, she panicked in fear that he would discover the layer of latex holding her flesh together. His hand went up, she pushed it down, and this continued over and over again. He thought she was just being modest, and she was dying to go home with him but couldn't figure out how to get from here (encased) to there (naked) without the guy, who was all over her, noticing. Unfortunately, rather than be exposed, she gave up and fled for a cab. And, ladies, she never did get a chance with this dude again—a sad state of affairs all around. How unfortunate that she let her embarrassment get the best of her! Truth is, I imagine he would have laughed it off.

I have to admit I probably would have bailed too! Everybody knows there is no such thing as a perfect body, and yet we strive for Barbie-like "perfection" with these garments. If our quest is exposed, it's doubly embarrassing and feels desperate.

Not wanting to be found out is only one of the reasons I don't wear Spanx. The other is plain discomfort. Even for my second wedding at age forty-five (if that isn't an occasion designed for marketing Spanx, what is?), I tried but failed. It's a dismal paradox. You feel ashamed because you aren't wearing Spanx and also because you are wearing them! Anyway, I ripped them off moments after squeezing into them and well before the photographer arrived. It's not worth it to me to feel so constrained. I relate to Liz Lange, the maternity fashion diva, who said, "I know I'm in the extreme minority, but I just can't wear anything like this—even tights in the winter: too itchy, too constricting." Same here; I hate tights.

Is a little smoothing worth feeling like a walking sausage? For the millions of women who swear by them, yes. They've made the company's founder, Sarah Blakely, a billionaire. That's nine zeros for something dreamed up from cutoff pantyhose. Many women say that they even double up. Supposedly, twice the Spanx makes for an even leaner silhouette.

From a 2016 *New York Times* article by Woolfer Judith Newman:

> Aviva Drescher, a former "Housewife" of New York, shared her best shapewear tip: "The secret to Spanx is double Spanx," She said. "You have to wear two at a time for serious sucking-in."

Diane Clehane is the Lunch columnist for Fish-bowlNY on Adweek's website, where each week she bears witness to "thousands of dollars of Spanx in one room" at the media hotspot Michael's.

"I can't imagine leaving the house in a dress without them," she said. "If they made one I could put over my head, I would."…

"How can you even be asking me this question?" shouted Jennifer Lupo, a New York lawyer who is to Rago Shapewear [a more girdle-like version of Spanx] what Anna Wintour is to sunglasses. "No woman should ever leave the house without Lycra on her thighs. I don't want to see my own cellulite, so why would I want to see yours?"

There is nothing revolutionary about Spanx and other shapewear. From whalebone corsets to fifties girdles to today's "body smoothers," women have believed that there was something unacceptable about their naturally shaped bodies for hundreds of years. What's really sad is when other women, such as Lupo, quoted in the *Times* article, project their own body shame onto others. Rather than critiquing other women's normal bodies, we could be looking to those with body confidence for inspiration. My friend Heidi once mused, "There are women out there who really don't care about their flab or pooch. Probably in Sweden, sitting in a sauna. Truly not caring."

As with so many issues for women over forty, do whatever the hell you want—if you enjoy being encased in Lycra, go for it. Me, I'd rather find a way to be more content with my jiggle. It's not likely to decrease, and I've lived too many years on this planet to be that uncomfortable. As for a thinner silhouette being more attractive, according to research done at the University of Iowa, heterosexual women consistently overestimate the value men attach to having a slender mate. What men are looking for is love—and to be able to get up our skirts—however that may occur.

THE GENIUS OF PERIOD PANTIES

We're so lucky to live in an age where menstruation is suddenly trendy. In the spring of 2016, a New York City pop-up shop opened (to crowds lining up around the block) called the Period Shop, where women could buy all things period related: cute undies, tampons, pads, chocolate bars, Midol, pajama pants, liners, you name it. Plastered on the subway are lascivious ads (suggestive fruit, sophisticated-looking women) for Thinx panties, with the tagline "Underwear for Women with Periods." It's a bit of a bummer that these developments are happening just as my period is on the wane, but never mind! Always happy to embrace a feminist trend, I rose to the occasion and promptly ordered Thinx online for my daughters. They seem to be a wondrous thing. You wear them instead of tampons or pads and the blood gets absorbed somewhere in the crotch and then washes away, leaving no stains! Hallelujah for women everywhere!

If your period is gone, Thinx's big-sister brand Icon could be the magic bullet for incontinence. Peeing yourself is a secret rarely passed down through the generations like a delicious apple pie recipe. According to a study by the University of California, Davis, 68 percent of women over forty experience leakage at least once a month. And nobody talks about it! Why? Because it's humiliating and made all the more so by our silence. Lead researcher Elaine Waetjen, MD, says that the fear of peeing oneself causes some women to avoid travel or attending social events. "There's embarrassment," she adds. "Some of my patients come to me and say they didn't feel comfortable talking to a male physician. Sometimes people were never asked. Some think it's such a normal consequence of having children and getting older that it's something they have to live with." (Read more about the betrayal of the bladder in chapter seven.) Forget extra-strength maxipads or the dreaded adult diapers Depends; modern technology is finally doing something to make women's genital lives a little easier.

SUMMER'S HERE AND THE WATER'S WARM

Oh, how I regret not having worn
a bikini for the entire year I was twenty-six.
If anyone young is reading this, go, right this minute,
put on a bikini, and don't take it off until you're thirty-four.
—NORA EPHRON, *I FEEL BAD ABOUT MY NECK*

AS USUAL, NORA WAS SPOT ON. If we had only known how luscious we were when we were younger, we could have spent so much less time agonizing over our bodies and so much more time conquering the world. I remember, on my first honeymoon in the Caribbean at the ripe age of twenty-three, spending no less than half the week agonizing about how fat I felt in my J.Crew shorts. Wow! What a fool I was, and how early it starts. According to research by *The American Journal of Maternal/Child Nursing*, 80 percent of ten-year-old girls believe they are fat and suffer from poor body image, kicking off a negative mind-set that harms overall self-esteem throughout the teenage years and well beyond. I now look back at those photographs of my younger self and marvel at my beauty. If only this imperative to appreciate ourselves through every phase of our lives were something that we could really convey to our daughters! We know now that it truly doesn't matter if we were flat, busty, chubby, skinny—in our teens and twenties we were also the pink of perfection, limber limbed and gorgeous. And if we were being generous with ourselves, we'd realize that the same is true now! In ten years we'll look back at some photo we cringe over today and think, "Damn, what a knockout." Same goes for ten years after that. So, Jesus—when do we just say, "Enough is enough. I'm good now. This is good"?

KATHERINE: *When my great-aunt Helen was 100 (she lived to 102), she said, "Oh to be 90 again." I think of this often as I struggle with time, its uni-directionality, its finitude, its casualties.*

Empowerment talk aside, bathing suit shopping is not for wimps— I'll give you that. Definitely low on the list of things I look forward to doing. I find it hard, and have since I became a teen. The situation isn't much better for girls today. *Discovery Girls*, a magazine for elementary school girls, recently drew a firestorm of criticism for its feature offering tips for finding the best bathing suit for your body type. It included suggestions for girls who are "curvy up top," "straight up and down," and "rounder in the middle." Ugh. The backlash was fierce but too late; the issue had already been sent out to nine hundred thousand tweens.

There are some bright spots, such as the online retailer ModCloth using its staff to model its swimsuit collection. Target has featured plus-sized models and in 2016 launched a "body positive swimsuit campaign" on social media, #NOFOMO ("no fear of missing out," for those of you, like me, who are slow on hip acronyms), encouraging real women to proudly post bikini pics. A couple of years ago, *Sports Illustrated* also jumped on the bandwagon, including Nicola Graham, fifty-six, in its annual bathing suit issue. Time will tell if these efforts are a lasting trend or simply marketing plans that will go in and out of favor depending on what sells.

Meanwhile, there is bathing suit shopping. Who was the sadist who designed the average department or sporting goods store swimsuit section dressing rooms? There are exceptions, like the high-end bathing suit designer Malia Mills, who has consciously created lovely, comfortable shopping oases bathed in natural light (and also features women of many shades, shapes, and ages on her website), but the typical experience is like stripping down in a fluorescent-lit coffin—one that is lined with a funhouse mirror. You will never, ever look as good in any suit you try on in that space as you will when you are actually having a wonderful time on the beach or by the pool, and the shopping experience can really ruin a whole day, or even the whole week in the wrong hormonal phase.

But there is a better way. This is how I like to do it when I realize the only suit I love is pilling and sheer enough to reveal my butt crack: I power up my laptop, find a friendly swimwear purveyor who offers free shipping and free returns (there are so many, from Zappos, which carries the famed La Blanca suit, to Gottex on Amazon, to Swimsuitsforall.com, which carries larger sizes), and purchase at least five bathing suits. Don't forget to read the sizing details carefully. Over the years, retailers have tried to flatter women by making clothing sizes bigger (oh my God, I'm a two!), while most bathing suit manufacturers have retained semitraditional sizing (oh my God, I'm a sixteen!). Ordering hundreds of dollars' worth of spandex online can feel nerve-racking, but repeat after me: "Free shipping and free returns." Just don't pull off that skanky sanitary crotch strip! When the box arrives, all you'll need is a full-length mirror, a glass of wine, and candlelight. It takes a little creativity, but you can turn what can be a daunting experience into one that's fun and sensual.

PLAN B

WHEN CONSIDERING SUMMER ATTIRE, we may reach a moment when the bikini feels too daunting. Or even the one-piece. And we may still bounce back from that moment to try again. But when feeling insecure, be kind to yourself. There are still choices. There's the skirted bathing suit route—not for everyone, but always an option, and one I embraced a few times postpartum.

For whatever reason, at this moment in my life a skirted suit screams, *"I give up! I am old!"* So I'm recommending Plan B, "Embrace the Caftan." Sometime back, writer Veronique Hyland wrote a perfect little piece in *New York* magazine called "How to Get Your Body Caftan-Ready for Summer." You get the idea: screw torturing yourself to get "bikini ready" in twenty-one days. Forget trying to look like your daughters in their bathing suits. It's not going to work anyway. Live your life, enjoy yourself, and go shopping (I love Calypso and Plume Collection) for a badass caftan, or ten!

Hyland claims that on the West Coast, caftan parties are all the rage and that actress Christina Hendricks is leading the charge. Whether true or invented, this is a trend I can really ride with abandon.

These are Hyland's steps (and every one but the first is highly optional):

1. Select a caftan of your chosen gauge and length. Stroke its gauzy fabric and whisper into its folds.
2. Let your flesh settle into the crevices of your comfortable, comfortable caftan.
3. Crumbs? Let them fall where they may, swaddled in your caftan.
4. Throw out your razor.
5. Throw out your bra.
6. Throw out the aloe vera lotion you bought last summer. You will not be getting sunburned this summer.
7. Release your inhibitions. Feel the rain on your skin.

We've talked about swimsuits, cover-ups, shoes, underpinnings—everything but the actual clothes. When it comes to midlife fashion, these are the easy things, the peripheral items we actually play around with. The basics—the pants, the skirts, the dresses, the jeans, the coats—are harder and very individual. Speaking with the the *Wall Street Journal* about why women's apparel spending decreases in mid-life, Gretchen Pace, general manager of Neiman Marcus in Beverly Hills, notes that mature women are a prime opportunity for retailers. "It isn't that women over forty-five don't want to shop anymore," Ms. Pace says. "It just isn't easy."

What we need to remember is that this is a phase, and a tricky one. This period of transition—psychological, physical, emotional—is profound, and we are finding our way to a new identity, almost a com-ing-of-age like the one we went through as teenagers.

Simplicity might help. Any good fashion guide will tell you, and probably more so as you age, that one trick is to find some basics that you love and stick with them. I've noticed I've become way less pre-occupied by trends and in many ways fret less about actual clothing items than younger women do. And my closet is no longer clogged with cheap fast-fashion items that have a shelf life of less than six months. "Chic is not a young girl's game," says Veronica Webb, the model and actress, who is fifty-two. "It's something that is acquired not with money, but with time and trial and error."

BLISS: *I fear appearing as if I'm clinging to my youth by wearing clothes or hairstyles or makeup that would better suit a younger woman. I think age is as much about a state of mind and a posture of being in your body as about how many wrinkles and rolls you have.*

My mom is seventy-eight and still dances and performs regularly, and her body is erect, graceful, and vital. But she doesn't like to wear certain things that she used to wear—tighter jeans, above-the-knee skirts, low necklines, and I don't think it's about some self-consciousness that she doesn't look good in those things, but more as if she would appear to be betraying the age and person she really is. I wrestle now when sometimes putting on things that feel more appropriate for a woman in her twenties or thirties between thinking, screw that, I'll wear what I want, and also that it's okay to dress my age.

Personally I have two lists, one of items I desperately hope to avoid (but probably won't be able to; let's be real), and the other my coveted basics that I'll cling to as I go gray and become infirm.

YOU GO, GIRL, BUT PLEASE NOT IN THESE

THERE ARE PLENTY OF WOMEN, and women I admire, who would say that there's nothing we can't wear as we age. They say, "Fuck anyone telling us what to do; I'll do what I want." This is a concept I embrace in principle, but perhaps not always in practice. There are, indeed, *for me,* some types of clothing and accessories that I dearly hope I'll never resort to, and particularly all at once, God forbid. These are items that say to me, "Call me Aunt Francine now."

In other words, while I have nothing per se against these items, and even imagine I will wear them at some point in the future (or even already have—shhh, don't tell!), they nevertheless represent something upsetting to me. Something about getting older and no longer being sexy or relevant in the way I still want to be. It's the awareness that their presence on my body may signify an aging out of what I used to love to wear and, indeed, who I used to be.

I broached the subject of "what not to wear" in a post to the group and was nearly knocked over and left for dead by the force of everyone's opinions. The comments cascaded over one another, "No muumuus and Birkenstocks," being drowned out by "But I'm wearing a muumuu and Birkenstocks!" Some ladies eschewed fuchsia, others teal. A brand loved by one was despised by another. And it was all in good fun, not about what another person should wear but what each one of us avoided because she equated it with being shunted out to pasture.

HEATHER: *I'll no longer wear the weight of the world on my shoulders. I tried it on when I was younger and it did nothing for me.*

Women's choices about what to wear are loaded with memory and cultural meaning. When we are younger we may get dressed to seek attention (or escape from it), to be provocative, to rebel. My middle-aged friends' biases ranged from what is and is not considered "age appropriate," to what was popular in the stifling hometown escaped at age seventeen, to how the movies depict "batty old ladies." Making your own list may seem a little silly, but it actually helped many of us to lighten our emotional baggage and loosen our self-imposed rules.

TEN THINGS I HOPE TO NEVER WEAR

HERE GOES, MY LIST. I made it for myself, and I'm sure it will change as I age, but it made me feel good. It helps me now, as my sense of self is shifting and I'm passing from one phase of life to another, to be clear about my preferences.

Remember, it is tongue firmly in cheek, because you should wear whatever the heck you want. We all know that you look fabulous if you feel fabulous, and I have no skin in the game of other women's choices.

1. **Eileen Fisher (and Chico's and Talbots and Lands' End).** A number of years ago, my best friend and I were musing about what we'd wear when we were "old." We settled on Eileen Fisher but assured each other that would be in the far distant future. (Joke's on us; here we are already!) "Am I ready for Eileen Fisher?" became our code for "Is it time to scrap my whole style/ wardrobe?" Don't get me wrong: I think head-to-toe Eileen Fisher can look fabulous on a five-foot-ten master triathlete or a dimpled pixie art gallery owner with stunning silver hair. I

own a gold-colored fifteen-year-old sateen quilt by Eileen that remains among my most prized bedding, and a couple of pieces of her clothing. But relying on head-to-toe sack clothing makes me feel like I have something to hide.

2. **Chunky accessories.** Last summer I took a trip to Maine and in Kennebunkport wandered into a lovely little shop that looked from the outside like a flower boutique. It turned out, inside, to be cornucopia of midlife/later-life accessories. The proprietor, a lovely woman in her late seventies, had gorgeous white hair in a small bun on the top of her head. She was swathed in flowing purple linen and reminded me (in a good way) of Mrs. Piggle-Wiggle. Her store was literally sagging under the weight of her merchandise. On every surface—everywhere!—there were gigantic necklaces and earrings, and rainbow-hued scarves and pleather purses in bright colors. There were fake pearls the size of jawbreakers, huge chunks of amethyst hanging from inch-wide chain links. I felt like an elf in a jewelry store; absolutely everything was oversized. I realized, after walking around in a stupor for a few minutes, that this is a certain kind of place that a certain kind of woman would adore. Not me. I'm not saying this jewelry is ugly; I'm saying for me it's like screaming, "I'm trying to distract from my changing face."

3. **Bright-colored reading glasses.** I try these on occasionally (again, is the idea to distract from our wrinkles?), and if my teenage daughters are with me, they shudder and say, "Please, no!" But they are awfully cute, and I do love purple...

4. **Birkenstocks.** Like birds migrating en masse or sea turtles crawling onto the beach to nest, there was a spontaneous mystery moment when women everywhere apparently made a tacit pact: Birkenstocks are the new stilettos. The German brand that touts its "tradition since 1774," as if that were a selling point, responded by producing sandals with racy colors, metallics, and collaborations with upscale stores like Barneys, but still, let's not kid ourselves. Flat, triangular plates lashed to your bunioned tootsies with wide leather straps are comfy, but not a hot look. I've owned the occasional chic silver 'Stocks over the years, but I dread becoming the woman who wears them every day. The way they make my toes spread makes me feel like eating granola and taking up macramé.

5. **Head-to-toe black.** Unless you are part of a coven. On second thought, that would be awesome. Joking aside, we all wear head-to-toe black sometimes, because it's easy, but as a "look" it seems dour at this stage of life and I'm veering away from it (which is very frustrating because it used to work just fine—why is that?!).

6. **Turtlenecks.** A hotly debated clothing item with powerhouse icons like Diane Keaton, Nora Ephron, and Diane Sawyer on the pro side. They make some women feel safe and cozy and camouflaged; they make me feel as if I'm getting hives. Also, as I age I think they accentuate my sagging neck, which might not be the desired look. I'm more of a Helen Mirren wannabe myself—as long as I have breasts, I might as well show some cleavage.

7. **Mom jeans.** The hipster girls scouring the racks of the Salvation Army for vintage high-waisted Lees are wrong and Tina Fey is right (as usual). However, praise be the demise of the ultralow jean and the comeback of the midrise with a hint of stretch. (See the next list, "Ten Staples I Hope Will Take Me a Long Way.")
8. **Crocs.** Of all the things on my list, I would hope that we are at least all in agreement on the hideousness of Crocs. Unless you are wading in a body of water or mud or are Mario Batali, no one over the age of ten should wear these things.
9. **Fanny packs.** They seem like a relic of days gone by, but I think my aunt Francine still wears one when she comes to visit us here in New York City. Not me, please.
10. This is actually not one thing I fear, but a plethora of clothing items I would rather avoid as I become "more mature" but don't even seriously think I'd ever entertain: **Velour tracksuits, UGGs, red hats, shoulder pads, pleated khakis**. I wanted to put "beaded eyeglass chains" here, but the truth is, I already have one.

All this said, here's the crux of the problem: What are the chic choices? We're caught between a rock and a hard place. We don't want to feel like we've given up, but we also don't want to look like we're desperately clinging to our youth. We avoid certain items that trigger self-censorship and shame by conjuring old-school sexist phrases like "mutton dressed as lamb" and new-school sexist phrases like "1661" (when a woman looks sixteen from the back and sixty-one from the front).

My friend Anne, who has long blond hair, jokes, "I swear, men have nearly fallen off their bicycles in a *Twilight Zone* mind bend after riding past me and realizing the babe that they just ogled could be their mother." She says it doesn't sting because—guess what?—she doesn't care about being desirable to a twenty-year-old boy. But it is emblematic of the fact that our culture still doesn't know what to make of women who are neither very young nor very old, especially ones who don't conform to certain expectations.

During the 2016 Academy Awards, costume designer Jenny Beavan received an Oscar for her work on *Mad Max: Fury Road*. When she mounted the stage wearing a leather motorcycle jacket, loose black blouse, cool tribal jewelry, and trousers, the gilded audience of Hollywood glitterati was deafeningly silent. Cameras caught some spectators glowering and others giggling. Stephen Fry, while hosting the BAFTAs, referred to her as a "bag lady." Beavan brilliantly shrugged off the incident, telling a reporter, "You've seen me. I'm short, I'm fat. I really would look ridiculous in a gown. What I was wearing at the Oscars was an homage to Mad Max—a kind of biker outfit." She added, "The only thing I would like is for my outfit to have a positive effect on what women feel about themselves. You don't actually have to look like a supermodel to be successful. If that could be a takeaway, I think that would be a good thing." Brava and perfectly spoken by a woman who snagged an Oscar designing costumes for a film about a renegade warrior woman and a matriarchal biker gang of seed-storing crones who save the world from a demented patriarchal despot.

Fashion and style are perhaps trivial compared to some of the other challenges we face, but what we wear and how we are perceived by the world is tightly wound up with status and self-esteem. It behooves us women to define ourselves. We certainly don't want to let anybody else do it for us.

TEN STAPLES I HOPE WILL TAKE ME A LONG WAY

*I get ideas about what's essential
when packing my suitcase.*
—DIANE VON FURSTENBERG

YOU AND ME BOTH, GIRL. These are my desert island clothes. The items I would pack into an overnight bag if forced to abandon the rest of my wardrobe. My list is so simple as to be incredibly dull. Yours may have gauchos or spangled shawls. Whatever it is, own it!

1. **Jeans.** As painful as it can be to go shopping for jeans. (I'm always terrified I'm going to need my husband's size. I know it's irrational, but that's some sort of Rubicon to me.) I can never pull skinny jeans all the way up, and low-rise jeans are dicey when you have a muffin top. But you really can find a decent, flattering pair of jeans to wear with basically everything, although it takes some bravery and persistence. Once you own them, you'll be grateful for them every day. Since you don't

have to bow to jean trends, go for it and get two pairs of the same style.

2. **A denim skirt.** The girly, dressed-up version of jeans. I love a straight one to just above the knee, and my current favorite buttons up the front. But long ones, flared ones, wraps, they are all good.

3. **Short-sleeve black cotton crewneck T-shirts.** They are flattering with the right bra, dressy with a necklace. The epitome of simple and chic.

4. **A couple of high-quality cashmere sweaters.** Both of my faves are slightly oversized, one crewneck and one V-neck, one gray and one black, and I wear them all the time with everything.

5. **Wedges.** However high or low you like, but I think a wedge is almost always sexy. I like them high, and even though I will one day break my ankle, I persist!

6. **Clogs.** As discussed. Love a clog! The more the merrier.

7. **Pajamas and lingerie.** We've already established that, for me, a bit of lace and silk feels sexy, whether worn for sleep only or peeking out of a top during the day.

8. **Simple gold jewelry.** Just some nice hoops and a long necklace; no need to get too funky or chunky.

9. **A glam pair of sunglasses.** I like to go a little big and movie star–ish. Especially useful on dog walks when I haven't had enough sleep.

10. **A chic wool coat.** For me this means long with a wrap sort of belt and luxurious material you can fold in around your neck.

A good coat is like a suit of armor that you can throw over anything and head into your day with confidence.

The point is not to have *my* list of staples but for you to figure out your own. What do you know you feel fantastic in? What would you pack into a single carry-on? I believe there is little point in wearing clothes that make you self-conscious, whether or not they are considered by others to be "tasteful" or "age appropriate" or whatever the fuck. Mindfully cultivating an attitude of not caring about what others think is very different from "giving up."

Find some style role models and keep them in mind as you traverse this aging continuum. They are out there! Are you, like me, inspired by Helen Mirren? Or Robin Wright in *House of Cards*? Julia Louis-Dreyfus in *Veep*. Michelle Obama, Holly Hunter, Parker Posey, Kim Cattrall! These are mine; who are yours?

Fifty-four-year-old Sophie Fontanel is a French journalist who has become a middle-aged style sensation. She posts daily fashion selfies on Instagram and now has more than sixty thousand followers. Among her many fashion tips (buy vintage, think about contrasting proportions, get comfortable taking selfies—love yourself!), this is my favorite:

> If you are obsessing at my age of being sexy, you will suffer a lot, because there are a lot of younger women everywhere, at any time. I think instead of putting yourself in competition with the younger woman, you

have to just find the way you appeal and it can be very, very invisible.

An interesting twist on the concept of becoming invisible, don't you think?

Ultimately, fashion in the second half of our lives is as much about feeling good as about looking good. Woolfer Kristen said, "I thought I would never wear a brooch. Then the other day I did. On a sleek modern dress, I wore the brooch of my late mother-in-law to express my wish for her to be present at our nephew's wedding, and it worked. I felt so mature and so relieved that I now have the freedom to wear whatever I like whenever I like. This is the freedom that comes with 'being over the hump.' It's definitely not all bad." Like white before Memorial Day, sartorial rules are made to be broken if you feel awesome. Never say never. If you feel like going to the grocery store in your pajamas, who's going to stop you?

I leave you with this:

> Elegance is not the prerogative of those who have just escaped from adolescence, but of those who have already taken possession of their future.
> —COCO CHANEL

CHAPTER TWO

(SEX AND RELATIONSHIPS)

DATE NIGHT AT THE ORGY DOME

The older one grows, the more one likes indecency.
—VIRGINIA WOOLF

STOP, HOLD THE PRESSES! Science says older women still love having sex. When a recent survey by the University of Pittsburgh Medical Center found that more than 60 percent of women over sixty who are married or living with a partner reported higher sexual satisfaction than in their youth, there were ludicrous headlines around the world like, "Middle-Aged Women Can Enjoy Sex, Study Claims." The cultural myth that menopause shrivels us up is complete crap. (Well, we do get dry, but that can be dealt with; stay tuned.) I have a fifty-nine-year-old girlfriend who is dating a nineteen-year-old young man, and not so surprisingly, the sex is mind-blowing (okay, questionable on an ethical level, but ripe for fantasy), and another who is actively looking for a gigolo. When I organized a get-together for my girlfriends at the erotic toy store Babeland in SoHo, not one of us walked out empty-handed. The staff begged us to come again, and we did (!), I promise you that. The truth is that we all become sexual beings much earlier than commonly acknowledged (I remember humping a girlfriend "for practice" on sleepovers when I was eight, don't you?), and we remain sexual beings 'til the day we die.

What the study itself pointed out was that women in their forties who are experiencing perimenopause or menopause (as well as the myriad stresses of being a grown-up) may well hit a few potholes on the road to sexy town, but by fifty, we've discovered some alternative routes. I spoke to Holly Thomas, MD, the lead researcher, who chuckled a bit over the way the media framed her team's work. "While some women do have sexual problems—I don't want them to feel that's not normal—sex does not get worse for everyone." During interviews with women aged forty-five to sixty, she and her colleagues heard that for many, "Their self-confidence had improved, they were more comfortable in their own skin, they felt more ownership of their bodies." She also said the other factors that actually helped improve women's sex lives were feeling free to speak up about what works (and doesn't work) in the bedroom and better communication skills in general with their partners.

So, we're still horny, we still like sex—but that doesn't mean it isn't complicated. In principle, sex after forty is the best: we can't (or soon won't be able to) get pregnant, we've learned what our bodies respond to in bed, and we're in many ways more confident and less self-conscious as people than ever before. Unfortunately, on the other hand, there is often, and often at maddeningly unpredictable intervals, the reality of our crazy hormones and how they are screwing with our lives. A friend who started a new relationship before perimenopause was delightedly banging her boyfriend twice a day—until her hot flashes kicked in. Now she's desperate for a few nights a week in bed alone with a carton of takeout Chinese and Netflix.

There are days when I feel like an actual cougar, hungrier for sex than I ever have been at any other time in my life. And then there are days—sometimes weeks—when my vagina feels bored, dry, and totally disinterested.

I'm not alone here. Vaginal atrophy, also known clinically as atrophic vaginitis (aka dryness) is the change in your cooch that develops when your estrogen starts to plummet. Estrogen, which is produced by the ovaries, plays a vital role in keeping our vaginal tissues lubricated and healthy. (You may remember, if you have children and breastfed, that a similar thing happened then—estrogen dropped, vagina got dry, hair fell out, you felt like crap. Once your period came back, you felt better. This time, though, your period is not coming back...)

When I was forty-two I had to have a D&C (dilation and curettage, a procedure to remove tissue from inside the uterus, also commonly done after a miscarriage or abortion) to remove a uterine polyp, and when I saw the pathology report, I was thrilled to read that all the tissue was benign, but mortified to see a clinical diagnosis of "vaginal atrophy." What?! I felt fine, wasn't even dry yet. But that diagnosis, apparently, is quite normal for a woman in her early forties. You don't feel dried up, but it *is* happening! And it proceeds apace, until one day you might be having sex and feel a sudden agonizing pain, like there's a dagger up there instead of a cock. The medical term for this pain is "dyspareunia," and it's a problem in so many ways. For starters, something you used to enjoy is now physically painful. If sex doesn't feel good, you're likely to have less of it, but unfortunately, like any other muscle (think triceps), to keep your vagina supple you have to "use it or lose it." If you start to lose it, intercourse feels even worse. It can be a vicious cycle, but it's not an unbreakable one.

I was forty-seven before the pain hit. And so far it's happened to me only once. I went into full-on battle mode attacking this particular problem, and I suggest you do the same.

HOW TO GET YOUR JUICES BACK

WE SIMPLY AREN'T AS LUSH down there as we once were, so the first line of defense is extra moisture.

It can take a long time for women to figure out that something as simple and accessible as an $8 bottle of lubricant can make a huge difference to their sex lives. Take it from me: you don't have to be wet to be hot, seriously. Claire Cavanah, one of the founders of Babeland, is something of a lube expert. "It's the workhorse of the sex toy world," she told me. There are so many choices out there it can be confusing—silicone lubes, organic lubes, water-based lubes, flavored lubes, flavorless lubes, seaweed-based lubes—so she broke it down. "Water based is what people often opt for; it's inert and has no harmful chemicals." She explained that the downside is that it doesn't stay as wet as silicone. Silicone is ideal for prolonged penetration and is "a must for anal sex." (I find that it works wonders for hand jobs and feels good on my nipples.) However, silicone lube degrades the surface of silicone toys. For most women experiencing dryness, a hybrid lube with traces of silicone is the way to go; just wash it off any toys right away.

In addition to lubing up for sex, women our age need to be generally focused on ongoing bedewing (that's actually a term for "making wet"). There are tons of products out there. My current favorite is a Vagisil brand called ProHydrate, which I squirt up inside my vagina once or twice a week. It doesn't leak and is made with hyaluronic acid, the same stuff that's in a lot of the facial moisturizers I use. The CEO of Vagisil, Keech Combe-Shetty, told me they think of it "like Cialis for women. It doesn't leak, or smell, so no one even knows you're using anything," and you're suddenly as wet as a twenty-year-old. Some of my friends swear by Hyalo Gyn, which is another similar product—hormone-free and colorless, inserted every few days—but that one I find a little leaky. Replens is another popular brand. Like so many things, it's all about personal preference; what matters is that you do the research and find a product that helps you.

Lots of my girlfriends go the completely natural route and transform their lady bits into a regular tropical paradise with coconut oil. No doubt you've heard about all the benefits of coconut oil for your hair and skin and nails; what you may not know is that it's great for the vag. I find that if I take a shower at night and rub maybe half a teaspoon (I'm not scientific about it; I just scoop some up with my pointer and middle finger and go to town) of organic coconut oil way up inside my cooch, I get into bed with a spring in my step. While there haven't been any major studies specifically testing the safety of using coconut oil as a vaginal lubricant, gynecologists generally concur that it's a fine alternative to synthetics, unless you are using latex condoms (it may break down the rubber) or are trying to get pregnant (oils may reduce sperm motility). In a recent interview with *Shape* magazine, Jennifer Gunter, MD, an ob-gyn at Kaiser Permanente Medical Center in San Francisco, said, "In my practice, many women who experience vaginal dryness, have chemical sensitivities, or vulvar sensitivities report really liking it." Plus, my guy says that it tastes good.

Then there are the pharmaceuticals. Your doctor can give you a prescription for any number of products, including Vagifem (vaginal tablet), Estrace (cream), Neo-Estrone (cream), Premarin (cream), Estring (low-dose vaginal ring). I've tried Estrace, an estradiol vaginal cream, and it does work. The caution with all of these is that you're using topical estrogen, which may be fine but over the long haul could be worrisome in terms of cancer. Currently, the *International Journal of Women's Health* says there's a lot of data supporting the safety of topical estrogen use for up to a year. Dr. Holly Thomas, the "frigid-over-forty" debunker mentioned earlier, concurred. The possible side effects (nausea, vomiting, bloating, stomach pain, breast tenderness, headache, weight changes, vaginal itching or discharge, mood changes, breast lumps, or spotting or breakthrough bleeding) might give you pause, as with any drug.

There's also (as with all the peri- and menopausal symptoms) the option of full-on hormone treatment, either bioidentical or synthetic, discussed at greater length in chapter seven. Even so, for what it's worth, I'm on a low dose of bioidenticals, and my vagina still needs extra moisturizing attention to keep it as comfy and wet as I like.

In addition, the recommendations for supplemental estrogen of any kind are a moving target; always check with your gynecologist about the most up-to-date research. (See Notes and Resources for reputable organizations that will also help guide you.)

Medical intervention with lasers is the last and final route, which I, thank God, have not yet had to resort to, but some of my friends have, and I'm guessing it's only a matter of time for me as well. It's kind of like Botox for your lady bits. "Vaginal revitalization" (there are various names for the procedure; the "Mona Lisa Touch" is the most popular right now) consists of a laser wand being inserted into the vagina for about five minutes for three sessions. The treatment is supposed to increase blood flow and collagen production in order to eliminate dryness and improve elasticity. It's done in a doctor's office with topical anesthetic and is reported to be painless (although one friend said, "The day I need a laser up my vag is the day I become celibate"). Insurance doesn't cover the procedure and the first series of three will set you back between $2,000 and $3,000, with a recommended follow-up session performed annually.

Back when you were twenty-eight, or thirty-five, could you ever have imagined you'd one day be spending so much time and money on vaginal lubrication? I never even bought lube before I was forty, and now I stash tubes of it everywhere—like tweezers! But here we are, and I can't stress enough how important it is to deal with. I know a few women who can barely have intercourse at all anymore. I don't know if they let it go too long or if their hormones are really just much more viciously depleted than mine (so far), but this is a real health problem that middle-aged women have to contend with.

ALL LUBED UP AND NO PLACE TO GO

AS I WRITE THESE WORDS, I'm forty-seven and I get my period every two to three months. I have hot flashes, night sweats, and sleeplessness. And then sometimes I don't. It's the same with desire. Some days it's higher than ever, and then suddenly, poof, it goes MIA. Maybe the insomnia doesn't help, although I've always believed that the "I'm too tired for sex" excuse is sort of bullshit. If I'm truly turned on, it doesn't matter how tired I am.

So how do we rev ourselves up when it feels impossible to get going sexually?

- **Naps.** If you really are too tired all the time, please start taking some naps! According to the Study of Women's Health Across the Nation (SWAN), the longest-running and broadest investigation of women's health and aging, for a lot of women sleeplessness does significantly impact the physiological factors that blunt libido. Make sleep a bigger priority. My hubby and I often take naps on weekend afternoons. We shower and get into bed naked, and whether we sleep or fuck, it's definitely sexy.

- **Weed.** Smoke a hit of weed before bed. But be warned: marijuana today is not what it was back when we were in tenth grade. For starters, you no longer smoke a whole joint! Today's pot will get you very high with one or two puffs, and many women I know claim that a hit before bed really sets the tone. Also, there are so many products out there: marijuana ghee for baking that you can make at home! Cannabis lube! Tinctures that require only a few drops under the tongue! My friend Debbie swears it's "the best natural medicine for libido boost." She says, "It helps spark my interest, and also to make the switch in mind-set from day-to-day getting things done to gettin' down." Another friend reports, "I rarely smoke weed during the day—it makes me paranoid—but for sex, it's amazing. The best and longest orgasms I've ever had. I recommend trying it." Describing her vacation in Jamaica, Woolfer Julie posted, "I had my best orgasm ever with an ex-boyfriend after smoking pot. Have been trying to replicate ever since! I don't have a lot of experience but it made every inch of my body so incredibly sensitive. I hope to find partners who are just as interested in my pleasure as their own and won't be threatened about how we get there—within reason, lol." For me it's hit or miss; sometimes it's been great for sex and sometimes I just fall asleep, but, hey, it seems worth trying, right?

GHEE WHIZ

Making Marijuana Butter at Home
Ingredients for Ghee:

2 pounds unsalted butter

Making the Ghee:
1. Melt the butter in a pan or a double boiler at a low to medium temperature so that the butter is hot enough to boil.

2. A froth will form on the surface of the butter.
3. Skim the froth with a spoon.
4. Continue skimming until no more froth appears.
5. Store in an airtight container in the refrigerator.

Ingredients for Cannabis Ghee:
1 pound ghee
1 ounce finely ground cannabis*
*THE FINER THE POWDERED CANNABIS, THE BETTER THIS METHOD WILL WORK.

Making the Cannabis Ghee:
1. Melt the ghee in a double boiler and allow to come to a simmer.
2. Add the cannabis slowly, and stir often.
3. Simmer for an hour.
4. Strain with cheesecloth or a fine-mesh strainer, and allow to cool.
5. Store in an airtight container in the refrigerator or in smaller portions in the freezer.

Use about 1/2 teaspoon per serving, so, if you are baking 24 cookies, that would be 2 ounces. Wait at least an hour before eating more than one serving, since the effect can take at least that long to be felt. You can store smaller portions in the freezer for up to three months.

The good old sexy nightgown. This still works to make me feel hot. Something snug but comfortable that highlights my breasts (Cosabella makes great ones) or a vintage-y silk slip. Removal is optional. I used to feel sad for a friend who never took her bra off during sex, but now I get it. I wish that every lady felt confident about baring her naked bod, but if the trade-off is not having sex,

I'd say do whatever makes you feel comfortable. As another friend confessed, laughing, "I have tons of sex, just never on top."

- **Porn.** Turn on the TV or cuddle up with your laptop. I've not resorted to watching porn with my man, but I have girlfriends who swear by it. I did go through a phase this year of watching *The Girlfriend Experience* and masturbating to it, so does that count? Remember, whatever works. Be open. Life is short.

TRACY: I love porn for what it is. A quick mood enhancer/cognitive stimulant when I'm looking to get myself off. Sounds harsh, perhaps, but at this age, I'm pretty much comfortable in my sexuality to speak frankly about it. However, I never watch porn while engaging in sex with my partner and don't feel that I need it. I just like it for me. YouPorn and Pornhub provide free porn with lots to choose from . . . There is always a little something for everyone!

- **Wellbutrin.** A lot of antidepressants kill your libido, but Wellbutrin can actually enhance it. Some doctors will prescribe it off-label to women with low sex drives. Not only can it make you hornier; it might even help you lose weight! Why am I not on it?

- **Bioidenticals and hormone replacement therapy.** We always get back here, don't we? As discussed in great detail in chapter seven, these hormones will definitely make you feel more like your old self; it's just a matter of whether you feel comfortable taking hormones, and when to start and when to stop. As I've said, I'm on them now, and they are my friends, but I also know women who have gotten breast lumps and decided to stop, or who drew the line at a certain age. Once you're off them, you do go back to square one.

- **Erotica.** Stimulating basics for your bedroom bookshelf: Nancy Friday's *My Secret Garden*, Anaïs Nin's *Delta of Venus*, anything by Susie Bright, the infamous *Story of O*, and a Victorian hottie called *The Pearl*. From there, you might move on to Literotica .com, an adult website with user-generated erotic fiction and fantasy. One of my girlfriends reads erotica aloud to her partner on long car trips. She swears by the results on arrival.

- **Novelty.** Have sex in a new place in the house or at a different time of day. I'm constantly wishing my husband would just take me in the kitchen or even on the couch. Doing it in bed all the time gets dull. Trying out positions or acting on a fantasy can help you find new ways to experience pleasure. Claire Cavanah, co-owner of the sex shop Babeland, says, "It can be challenging if you've had sex one way for a long time and now it's not working. Reassess what turns you on and give yourself permission to pursue pleasure."

- **Short-term abstinence.** Limit a session to kissing or oral or hand jobs, or masturbate in front of each other.

■ **Sex date.** "Date night" gets a big sigh from lots of people, and I get it. My first husband literally ran from the room every time it was uttered, but then, he's now my ex. The fact is, sometimes we just need to plan sex. Sometimes we need to go for it when we are not in the mood, just because it's been too long. Remember: *Use it or lose it*. Keep saying that to yourself. Would you rather be closed for business? I doubt that. Getting ready and knowing sex is on the books can be an aphrodisiac.

■ **Vibrators.** Everyone has them these days, and read on for my own tale on toys.

■ **Addyi** (flibanserin, the "female Viagra"). Although the FDA approved the pill's use for hypoactive sexual desire disorder (HSDD)—in other words, low libido—in 2015, the jury is still out on the drug's safety and effectiveness. One big drawback is that it can cause dangerously low blood pressure, especially when combined with alcohol, so forget that warm-up cocktail.

■ **Polyamory anyone?** Have a frank talk with your partner about opening up your relationship. One friend recently told me that she thinks polyamory is going to be the next big civil rights movement. That may be a bit of an exaggeration, but it certainly seems more mainstream now. Could there be a version of this— swapping, sex parties—that might work for you? I think I'm too jealous, but I do love the idea…

- **Role-playing.** A between-marriages boyfriend of mine once suggested we meet at a bar and pretend to be sexy strangers. I became a thirty-two-year-old single teacher, which was bizarrely unimaginative, even for me, but the resulting sex was still super-hot.

- **Sexting.** Have you ever sent your guy a picture of your breast? You probably have; I haven't. But maybe it's time. It's *very* common and might add a spark.

Then there are toys and kink, and other adventures...

DESPERATE MEASURES

I HATE TO BE THE BEARER of more bad news, but here goes: as we age, the clitoris can become less sensitive. Since the majority of women require clitoral stimulation to climax, this is truly a bummer, but again, not the end of the world. The mechanisms of sexual response are complex, but a couple of reasons related to this change are reduced blood flow in the genitals and depleted hormones. If you have a hard time reaching orgasm without major clitoral stimulation, here are two tips:

DO:
The Hitachi Magic Wand is the mother of all vibrators. It's not pretty and is about as big and heavy as a baseball bat (good luck getting it

through airport security!), but it gets the job done. Remember to lube up! Woolfer Gina is adamant about hers: "I don't want to live in a world where this magic wand isn't permitted. A penis and a tongue are great, but frankly they don't always have the finishing touch (when they do, it's great), nor are they always available for this divorcée, who sometimes has a relationship, and sometimes does not. Further, as I get older, I just need more pressure and focus. It doesn't have anything to do with my man. I'm used to having intense orgasms and whatever I need to do to keep them alive and well, I will."

DON'T:

"Scream Cream"—I was tipped off to this idea and went on a hunt, but this stuff seems to be a bit of a unicorn. It's prescribed off-label, for application to the clitoris, and contains a host of hard-core amino acids and hormones to loosen your libido, but my doctor worries it's not so safe and she wouldn't even give me a script for research purposes!

IN THE MOOD, BUT NOW WHAT?

ALL THIS TALK ABOUT VAGINAL DRYNESS and how to get in the mood can be a total buzzkill, but now that you have some options, let's move on to the fun stuff. One of the absolute best things about getting older for me is a complete lack of discomfort around all things sexual. In my twenties or thirties when I wanted to talk about sex with a partner, I was always too shy to directly say what I meant or ask for what I wanted. And I'm not a shy type. But I would bury my head in the pillow or giggle. That all seems to have gone the way of my perky tits—in other words, out the window. Now I love to talk about sex with my partner. In fact, I love to talk about things that I don't even want to do, like golden showers or getting a pearl necklace or getting fucked in my butt (see the section on anal sex in a few more pages!). I find the language titillating and I like being playful about it.

That said, I've come to realize I'm clearly from an older generation regarding sex. I was born in 1969! I read about millennials taking Molly and having sex with one another in a big pile, or twentysomethings going wild on Tinder, with a new guy every night, and all this makes me feel a bit weary. One middle-aged man I know told me that he dated a twentysomething who wanted to pee on him and use equipment involving straps, chains, and dildos. How many women over forty had heard the term "pegging" until we learned about it from *Broad City*? If the hype about what all these youngsters are up to is even half true, I say, God bless.

I was sexually active from the age of fourteen and am far from a prude, but I have to admit that my forays into anything outré were slow in coming (so to speak, ha-ha). And I'm actually grateful that I grew up before Internet porn, with all its gymnastic stunts and plasticized bodies, was just a click away, and that I discovered what I liked in bed through curiosity and experimentation.

My first serious boyfriend, a football player named Earl, gave me sweet orgasms with his fingers while we fooled around on the carpeted floor in his basement TV room. It never occurred to me to masturbate (I have no idea why) and what Earl did to me was enough. I was nineteen the first time I did play with myself, a good five years after I'd lost my virginity. It was in my childhood bedroom and it was a few weeks after my mother had died. Michael, my boyfriend at the time, had gone away on a trip, and I remember the gray light of morning as I used a pillow between my legs and climaxed. It almost seemed like an accident.

Good sex is like good bridge. If you don't have a good partner, you'd better have a good hand.

—MAE WEST

Even after that, I swear I somehow forgot about masturbation as an option. In my twenties, a man I lived with was curious about sex toys, and unmarked brown boxes started arriving in the mail. He would gleefully pull contraptions out from under the bed, like a butterfly gizmo that was supposed to attach to my clit, or a vibrator that you could wear on your finger, and so forth. I was good-natured about the whole thing, but not particularly interested in all that flimsy, colorful plastic, and he soon gave up. In retrospect, I feel a little bad about that. I think I was self-conscious and had I been more courageous it might have been great fun—but it didn't appeal at the time.

That's a rather long way of saying it took me until the ripe old age of forty to appreciate the pleasures of masturbation and sex toys, and boy, have I embraced them with glee.

DANGEROUS EXES AND TAKING THINGS INTO YOUR OWN HANDS

IT STARTED WITH A POSTDIVORCE Match.com boyfriend—let's call him Simon—who wanted to tie me up and spank me, which, to my surprise, I liked. He had taken previous partners to sex parties and liked to swing, and I found his stories titillating. Simon's authority beckoned; I'm not sure how else to put it. As a working, divorced mom of four, it was a turn-on to let someone else be the boss. Sadly, it turned out that in addition to being sexy, Simon also had a paranoid, nasty streak, and I had to let him go before we got to explore further.

Another postdivorce boyfriend took me to a strip club while on vacation in Key West—I know, I'm sure you've all done this already, but for me it was new—and at first I was kind of mortified. I felt bad for the women dancing (subjugation!), and the men creeped me out (sleazeballs!). But a couple of drinks later, I relaxed into it and started to find the whole thing kind of exciting. Then a woman came on stage who, for whatever reason, appealed to me. She was blond and busty, with a sweet face, and when she asked if we wanted to go in a back room, we said sure. That lap dance, with my guy hard and leaning into me from behind and Ms. Stripper grinding in front of me, her breasts brushing up against mine, was one of the most erotic experiences I've ever had in my life. At age forty-two! When an orgasm is evading me, I still use the memory, and I know my ex, even though we are long broken up, uses it too.

Around that time, my girlfriend Bliss casually mentioned her vibrator, and it aroused my curiosity. Obviously I'd heard of vibrators before, even used them (remember the guy who liked getting them via the mailman), but this was different; suddenly it felt like an important concept and an item I could own for my own pleasure. Not long after dating Key West guy, I was waiting to pick up one of the kids from a playdate near the drag of hipster stores in Williamsburg one afternoon, and I wandered into a sex shop and bought a little purple thingie that soon became my new best friend. It looks like a halved egg wrapped in smooth purple latex with a busy little motor inside. As a starter toy, it was perfect: small enough to fit snugly in my right hand, soft to the touch but never flagging, and nimble enough for me to use while on my back, stomach, or side. Voilà, a convert was born!

I'm aware that masturbating regularly and owning one vibrator when you are forty is not exactly news—according to the *Journal of Sexuality*, about half of American women ages eighteen to sixty have at least one. But for me, better late than never! Now, nearing fifty, I have a drawer full of sex toys (I rotate between six or seven different vibrators depending on mood and situation) and some fur handcuffs I'm begging hubby number two to deploy.

SEX TOYS 101 FOR THE VIBRATOR VIRGIN

Walking into a sex shop when you have never used a toy can be fun, but it can also be intimidating. I asked Claire of Babeland fame for her advice, and here's what she says:

> To get started choosing a sex toy, think first about how you might want to use it and what kind of stimulation you

like. There are vibrators that are best for internal use and G-spot stimulation, external use for clitoral stimulation, and some are dual action and do everything all at once. Visiting a friendly store like Babeland lets you check out the options in person. You can pick them up, figure out how they work, and get a sense of what kind of vibration the toy has—thumpy, buzzy, et cetera—and what it feels like. If you can't physically go to a store, online sites have a lot of information and helpful customer service too. Read reviews and product descriptions to get a sense of the toy. At the end of the day, go with the one that turns you on, that makes you feel excited.

She offers these recommendations for the newbie:

- The classic Rabbit Habit is an example of a dual-action vibe. The ears deliver vibration to the clit while the shaft rotates and feels amazing on the G-spot.
- The We-Vibe's C-shape hugs the clit and the G-spot, operates with an app, and can be worn during sex for that extra oomph most women need during intercourse. This has been our bestselling style of couple's toy for years.
- Our most popular rechargeable vibrating cock ring is the Mio by Je Joue. It's comfortable and pleasurable for both partners, with customizable settings.
- The Crave Bullet is a discreet, powerful, rechargeable choice. Your clit will love it.
- Lovely, and curved for the G-spot, Lelo's Gigi 2 has multiple settings and patterns. This is one of our perennial favorites.
- For decades the Hitachi Magic Wand has set the standard for powerful vibrators and it's well deserved. This is a guaranteed orgasm every time.

Speaking of fifty-eight-year-old hubby number two, the man with whom I love to talk about sex...In the summer of 2016 we went to Burning Man and had what, as of this writing, was my biggest sexual adventure. On the third or fourth day, biking around in the hot desert, we passed the famous "orgy dome," a place we'd both heard about but never discussed. We stood, we stared, we felt uncomfortable, and then we rode on. But that night he kept bringing it up (as in "If we one day went to one of those sex tents") and it evolved into a kind of sexy, teasing conversation. Soon we found ourselves doing a little Internet research, and, boom, the next night we snuck away from our friends and headed over to the dome, with a clean sheet, some lube, and a little tequila stashed in our Camelback. Mind you, we had never even remotely considered doing anything like this back in New York; this was definitely a "we're not in Kansas anymore" moment.

As we waited on line (a *very* long line—we waited over two hours! to get into an orgy dome!), my man was visibly nervous. I felt pleased with myself, like I'd called his bluff and was being super-adventurous, and I tried not to think about what lay before us. Then we showed ID to prove our ages (forty-six and fifty-eight, hello!) and were ushered into a giant waiting tent, with other couples and groups sitting around staring at one another. Would we be having sex with these strangers soon?!

We'd read up, so we knew the gist of what lay before us. Visitors are asked a few questions about consent and told the basic rules: you have to disrobe in the ante-tent, where you are given a bucket to store your essentials (water, etc.), and the dome provides extra condoms and lube should you run short. Then you walk into the main area and enter the middle of the dome. You then have the option of going to "the left" or to "the right." "The right" is where no one can approach you, so it's a room full of people having sex in couples (or triples or however you come in together) on their own discrete piece of orgy-dome real estate (a futon, a couch). You can watch (although not stare), but you can't touch or approach anyone else. "The left" is more of what you might think of as an orgy. On the left, anyone can approach you and ask for your consent to do things to you, to get involved in what you are doing, to have things done to them.

The first guy who explained the rules to us was really chill, and we sort of just blankly nodded like the mortified newbies we were and said okay. When he walked away (we were still clothed at this point), we looked at each other like, "What the hell are we doing?!" but we just sat there until they called our number (as if we were casually buying sliced turkey at the deli counter), and then we had to walk to the next chamber, where we disrobed and left our clothes on a shelf. So, yes, now we were naked and being ushered along. Bucket, check. Then the entry to the main room. The big moment. This could have been disastrous, a moment of paralyzing fear, but a very suave maître d' of sorts approached us and asked what we'd like to do, go left or go right? We both shrugged and giggled nervously and were saved when he pointed out a newly vacant couch on the right, and we hustled our naked asses right over.

Okay, so the three things you have to know straight off are: (1) the place was super-clean, (2) the lighting was perfect, and (3) everyone was super-good-looking. And I was not stoned or drunk. It was a perfect night and the other orgy-goers were gorgeous. (They just were, it's true! Although I admit I had been living in an RV in the blazing desert for four days, so a hot dog might have looked gorgeous.) We whipped out our sheet and started having sex, right there in front of everyone else having sex, and I gotta tell you, it was awesome. We must have stayed for two hours. We had sex in various positions, did oral, and watched people do all sorts of things you can probably imagine. There were two women using a dildo, someone who was getting mildly spanked (as was I), and lots of regular, steamy sex in all sorts of positions.

Going "to the left," which is where anything can happen, has now become code in our relationship for that tantalizing thing we may never experience. But who knows? Only time will tell. My husband teases me because more than actually *doing* anything, I like to *talk* about doing things. Like maybe we should swing? I've looked into sex clubs and sex parties in New York but so far feel like it might just be too creepy, dirty, or unsafe. That said, five years ago if you had told me I'd go to an orgy dome in the middle of the Nevada desert, I would have called you crazy. Who knows how much more exploration I still may do?

I think the bottom line is, as super-sexy Lenny Kravitz says, "It ain't over 'til it's over." I'm doing things now I never did when I was younger, and I'm more comfortable about it than ever before. My breasts are sagging and he may not always be as hard as he once was, but sex can be as intimate and delicious as always and I imagine will stay that way for a long time to come.

ANAL, ANYONE?

AM I IMAGINING IT, OR has ass play in general gotten a lot more popular than when we were young? When I started dating after my divorce in my thirties, I could not believe how many men were trying to stick their fingers up my butt! A couple of years ago, minutes into the season opener of the HBO show *Girls,* uptight Marnie got rimmed, right on TV! I have to confess that I'm a chickenshit on this particular front. I've never put my finger in anyone's ass and doubt I ever will. I haven't attempted anal sex since George Bush's father was president. It always seemed painful, and I'm a bit of a poop prude, I admit it (I don't want those yucky bacteria in my vagina!).

Obviously, I'm no expert here. But I'm also not a killjoy, and I love that there are women who love it! Writer Toni Bentley is a notorious fan, and in her book *The Surrender,* she describes how being regularly sodomized for four years by a man whose name she never even knew was a life changer:

> And then he fucked me in the ass. Is this what he learned while out of town? It was the first time ever for me. Ever. My God, he was good. I mean bad. What nerve he had. So graceful. It was very slow, very careful, very connected and painful. It was in here, in there, that I first tasted the experience of moving through pain and fear to that plateau on the other side, where I met this man in a foreign land called Bliss.

Some women have told me that the intense part of anal sex is that it's an act of trust, that you submit to your partner, you literally stop being "tight ass" and allow yourself to be completely "open." That said, anal certainly doesn't have to hurt—quite the opposite. Bentley might have liked the pain with her pleasure, but that's her thing. If you are anal curious but a backdoor virgin, you might be interested to know that there are many more nerve endings around the anus than around the vagina. *Moregasm*, the fantastic guide to "mind-blowing sex" by the women who started the sex toy chainlet Babeland, advises to go slow and stop if you feel discomfort. You can start by experimenting with a finger or a small toy like a butt plug or beads (and a lot of silicone lube!). It goes without saying that you should wash thoroughly before any ass play and avoid transferring germs from the anus to the vagina by finger, toy, or penis. If your partner is game, make the most of all those sensitive nerve endings by rimming or light digital stimulation without penetration. Hmm…maybe I'll even go back to it.

HE'S JUST NOT THAT INTO YOU

You have to know that an older man cannot hang from a chandelier.
—DR. RUTH

THERE'S A LOT OF TALK at our age about vaginal dryness and dwindling libido, but what people don't discuss so much is male loss of desire. The first time I encountered a not-so-hard penis on a somewhat regular basis, I was shocked. Did he not want me? Was I not attractive to him? Many women I know who are out there dating report that limpish dicks are a widespread issue. Guys' hormones peter out too, you know! After age thirty, men's testosterone begins a gradual decline, which can cause erectile dysfunction (ED), loss of interest in sex, fatigue, depression, and overall muscle loss. So, it's not that he's not that into you: it's that his testosterone peaked *decades* ago. Alcoholism, liver disease, obesity, diabetes, and the use of certain drugs can also impact testosterone levels. There are many other causes of ED as well, from chronic diseases to emotional issues.

What not to do? If you're still hoping to get some, best not to shame him. Taking action to improve your sex life can be sensitive at best and it's no secret that men can be ultratouchy about their virility. Making a fuss and acting exasperated can definitely have the opposite effect from what you are seeking. I've heard of men suffering from prolonged impotence who claim it began when their partners harped on their unreliable members. So tread carefully, but tread you must. Saying nothing out of fear of confrontation or concern for his ego will only result in you both being unhappy. Frankly, I also see it as a feminist issue: there's nothing to be ashamed of in asking for what you need. You aren't saying he's deficient; you're saying that you both, as a couple, need to find some new solutions. Women have for far too long been told to be quiet about their sexual needs. Why should we be?

Consider this: by the time we hit forty-five, as many as one out of three women has had an abortion, nearly three-quarters have obtained some kind of medical birth control from a physician, and

80 percent of us will have given birth, not to mention the countless other medical procedures, interventions, pokings, and proddings our reproductive systems regularly endure. Typically, men at the same age have done almost nothing. Outside of buying condoms or lube, they have probably spent precious little money on their sexual health, nor have they been cut open, stitched back together, or taken a drug. Now might be the time, even though it could be a hard pill to swallow.

Men are less likely than women in general to go to the doctor, and they can be reluctant to take medicine. They might be ashamed to bring it up during a physical exam. Or maybe they are afraid of side effects, like heartburn or dizziness. (As reasonable as this is, we've had to deal with side effects from things like the Pill our entire lives, so, honestly, man up.) They can also (as unappealing as this is to visualize) still ejaculate with limp penises and are sometimes happy to just go that route. But if you're anything like me, and like a lot of my friends, you really want a hard cock. It makes us feel desired; it feels good inside us; sometimes we like to be pounded. It's sexy. Thus, the "honey, maybe you should see a doctor" conversation has to be had, and sometimes more than once. Checking testosterone levels is done by a simple blood test, and the doctor may refer your guy to a urologist for further treatment or prescribe an ED drug such as Viagra or Cialis.

A young woman in her twenties whom I met while I was working on this book asked me recently if I was "pro or con on ED drugs." This struck me as funny. Do I have a choice? If we need them, we need them, is how I see it.

My friend Jenny, whose partner uses them regularly, says it's no problem at all. He pops a Cialis on Friday nights and is pretty much good to go all weekend. During the week they tend to go au natural, which for this guy (in his late fifties) is hit or miss. He gets erect, but maybe not as hard as he once was, and it may not last as long. She's fine with that, and their intimacy might involve more oral sex, or just cuddling, when that's the case. But on the weekend, she gets what she wants, which is occasional hard penetration, and he seems to like it too.

I have heard some nightmares. One friend dated a guy with no prostate who had a shot he kept in his freezer. If Cialis didn't work he would give himself an injection in the ass and then be rock solid for about ten minutes. Quick! Another woman I know dated a guy who took Viagra regularly but never ejaculated. She felt like the sex never ended, which is not really what anyone wants. My girlfriend Cindy's husband is having trouble lately but he refuses to take drugs, says they give him headaches. Now their only physical contact is the sporadic hug or cuddle, and that's making her miserable.

The best advice about erections came, of course, from a Woolfer. Elisa says:

> Cock rings work wonders, but working toys into the mix is good to take the spotlight off the droopy party. Remember that part of your guy's lack of interest may well be his disappointment at his unreliable vigor. No matter how evolved he is, it's a depressing iden-tity shift/sign of mortality that is not easily shaken off. For a lot of men, the woman's pleasure becomes an even more interesting focus, which is why older

guys can be way more fun than young sex machines. Staying empathetic and playful (above all, not taking it personally) makes all the difference.

GOING HEAD TO HEAD: VIAGRA VS. CIALIS

Have you been contending with a sluggish penis lately? Consider yourself among friends. Although ED drugs rake in $4 billion a year for pharmaceutical companies, they are not as widely used as you might think. According to research by Harvard Medical School, nearly 50 percent of men ages forty to seventy have experienced some degree of erectile dysfunction, but only 7 percent have taken a drug for it. If your partner is one of the few, the proud, the brave, who is willing to try, here's what he should know about ED drugs.

1. Viagra, the most commonly prescribed drug in this category, is a one-shot deal. Take it and you have about four hours of prime erection time. Cialis is effective over about thirty-six hours.
2. Neither drug produces spontaneous erections. Both take between fifteen minutes and an hour to enter the bloodstream. At that point, do not expect to get a boner like the pop-up on a Butterball turkey. The meds don't work without sexual stimulation. So get busy with some foreplay (which is what most ladies want first anyway!).
3. ED drugs don't work for everyone. Some men with severe erectile dysfunction will not respond at all to these meds. For the rest, it often takes a few tries to get the timing right and take it the proper way (e.g., Viagra needs to be taken on an empty stomach). Many men get ED drugs from their GP, who may not have in-depth knowledge about how they work. Do your research and try to be patient.

---

4. If one drug doesn't work or has unpleasant side effects, you can try another. In addition to Viagra and Cialis, there are two other ED drugs, Stendra and Levitra (Staxyn), on the market.
5. Men with certain medical conditions such as a history of congestive heart failure, stroke, or low blood pressure should not take ED drugs. Each drug has its own side effects and potential for dangerous interactions with other medications. Talk to your doc.
6. They aren't free. Most insurance doesn't cover these medications. Viagra can cost up to $45 per pill. There is a lower-dose Cialis that can be taken daily (ideal for frequent and spontaneous nookie) that costs $9 per pill but must be taken at the same time every day (it adds up to a hefty $270 a month). You can find coupons and discounts or discuss getting higher doses (to split in half) with your physician in order to reduce the bill.

Sex comes in many forms and perhaps more so as we age. Erection-penetration-ejaculation may no longer be the hard-and-fast (forgive me) standard that it was when we were younger, but the trick is flexibility and communication.

Sexologist and sex educator Logan Levkoff told me that at our age, "Don't waste your time with things that aren't feeling satisfying. Move on and try something new." The mantra she recommends for any stage is, "There are no rules. The way we have been taught we are supposed to look and feel, those rules are bullshit. Your journey is yours alone and it might look different from your friend's or your sister's or anyone else's."

I know that for me and my partner, we generally go to sleep and wake up holding each other in some sort of sexual way—his hand cupping my breast, my hand gently gripping his balls, him rubbing my ass—and so I feel like we are sort sexually engaged most of the time, on one level or another. This kind of closeness feels good and is satisfying, and it doesn't require clockwork orgasms.

PLAYING FOR THE OTHER TEAM?

IF YOU'RE STRAIGHT, CAN YOU tell me how many times you've said you wish could just chuck all these men and hook up with a woman? Plenty, I'm sure. If only it were that simple. Not only heterosexual couples experience bumps with sex drives and expectations at this age. My friend Kayla tells me, "I've always been into sex. If anything I want it more, which is unfortunate because I get it less, as my partner Ellie is older and has experienced a declining libido coupled with the effects of antidepressants. We try to talk about it and deal with it and fix it, but sometimes we ignore it for way too long. Self-pleasure is awesome, but not exactly a solution."

And if you are in a same-sex relationship you might get to have a "doubly intense" ride on the hormone roller coaster, as my cousin Cynthia described it. But it can also be helpful to be with a woman who truly understands. "About two years ago I'd notice the bed was getting hot and sweaty in the night, and my wife would be complaining about how hot it is in the room and can we open a window and I'd be like, 'Um, you're having a hot flash.' It started as a joke until we realized, yes, that's actually exactly it!"

KEEPING YOUR LONG-TERM RELATIONSHIP HOT (AND OTHER OXYMORONS)

If she is one of the many women who have been fucked
when they wanted to be cuddled, given sex when what they
really wanted was tenderness and affection, the prospect of
more of the same until do death do her part from it is hardly
something to cheer about.
—GERMAINE GREER, *THE CHANGE: WOMEN, AGING AND THE MENOPAUSE*

LET'S SAY YOU'VE BEEN MARRIED or living with the same fellow for ten (twenty, thirty?) years, he's having trouble getting it up, and your love life is sputtering out. He pops a pill and it works like magic. Great, now he's got a rock-hard erection—but is that always a good thing? What if you've been suffering from insomnia and a dry vagina and your partner suddenly has a two-hour hard-on and is as randy as an eighteen-year-old? Being clear about what you both actually want out of your sex lives is crucial. Maybe regular intercourse isn't such a big deal to the two of you, and making out, touching, oral sex, or cuddling provides a satisfying connection. You won't know unless you talk about it.

Since I got divorced after sixteen years with husband number one, I can't speak to the ups and downs over decades of marriage. But that said, many of my friends are in that boat, as are huge numbers of Woolfers. Here's one moving take from a woman named Bonnie:

For the first couple years of marriage, passion was a cure-all, but once the dopamine rush subsided, we've had to discover so many strategies to simply tolerate each other's daily presence, let alone stay intimate and romantic. We're twenty-three years and counting.

I've had two epiphanies about long-term relationships, one about a decade ago and one very recently. They have become the talismans I turn over in my brain when we get into a pissy phase. The first realization was that if you are in a glowy, happy place in your marriage, it won't last forever, and if you are in a miserable, loathing place, that won't last forever either. It took many years to see the cycles and trust that we would pass through whatever it was and not despair.

The second is particularly important for this later phase of our marriage, now that it's just me and him in the proverbial empty nest. This year, when the last kid went to college, I was stuck on this unsettling image of the two of us staring silently at each other across the dinner table—forever. I wasn't swept up in an image of us riding a wave of adoration into our golden years. I was more like, "Can we start going on separate vacations now?"

One night I was cooking and listening to an interview with the philosopher Ruth Chang on how to make hard choices. She proposes that by taking ownership of hard decisions, you "become the author of your own life." I wanted to do a thought experiment about the concept...what choice could I make on the spot? "I'm going to choose having a happy marriage" popped into my head. I felt a little giddy. My husband ambled in at the exact moment dinner was ready (this usually bugs the crap out of me). I said, "Honey, I've made the choice to have a happy marriage." He beamed. "It only took you twenty years." So far, it's working, but of course (see epiphany number one), I know it won't last...

FOUR VERY SCIENTIFIC REASONS TO HAVE SEX

HERE'S A DIRTY LITTLE SECRET: sometimes I feel I'm just "done" with sex. Like dying your hair or wearing a bikini, it can feel like a chore that a grown woman is at liberty to dispense with. We can talk blithely about orgies, BDSM, rimming, toys, and on and on as if midlife were or could be one endless kinky birth-control-free fuckfest, but for a hundred reasons from stress to hot flashes to a yearning for genuine autonomy, having sex can lose our interest—for a short time or forever. In case you need convincing, there are some compelling reasons to keep on doing it:

1. It's good for your relationship. Sex can bring you closer to your partner. When you have sex, your brain releases oxytocin, the so-called love hormone. This neurotransmitter increases trust and bonding.
2. Orgasms can ease pain and fight depression. Again, due to the release of hormones, getting off either alone or with a partner can block pain and boost self-esteem. Sex has also been shown to reduce migraines because of the rush of blood from the head to the genitals.
3. Sex keeps your pelvic floor (PF) muscles in shape. Toned PF muscles can help prevent urinary incontinence. And keeping them strong triggers more powerful orgasms—which in turn strengthens PF muscles. One of Mother Nature's wonderful positive-feedback loops.
4. Sex is a soporific. You may feel too tired to have sex, but in fact, getting it on before bed can help knock you out and enhance your REM sleep.

But maybe you really, truly don't care to have sex—you would rather spend your time and energy on something else. You don't want to wash the sheets. Whatever. Our sex-sells media-driven society tells us that screwing is like eating and breathing—everybody is doing it all the time, or needs to be. Sure, as a species we are biologically compelled to reproduce, but that doesn't mean there's something intrinsically wrong with you if you don't want to do it.

Over dinner with a group of long-married girlfriends, a woman

I'll call Jane said, "I just don't feel right unless Paul and I have sex at least three times a week." This was a conversation stopper. Aside from newly (re)married me, none of the other women at the table was having sex with her spouse more than once a week, and one hadn't had any kind of sexual contact for a year.

There are a lot of reasons women in long-term relationships don't talk about their sex lives or lack thereof. We don't want to impugn our own seductiveness or suggest our partners aren't virile; we don't want people to judge our relationship as "loveless." But once women start opening up about frequency, it's clear there is no "normal." What I can say for sure is that a lack of spontaneous, insatiable desire is commonplace in long-term relationships and can sometimes feel like a huge bummer.

Early in a relationship, the release of neurotransmitters like dopamine stimulates the brain's reward and pleasure centers in much the same way as addictive drugs like cocaine. I was in that period a few years ago, when I met the man who became my second husband. God, was it delicious. I still love the feel of his skin and his hands on my body, but that first year or so I thought I would die from the pleasure. Alas, most research says that the sex high fades in between one and three years, and I guess that particularly heightened eroticism does have to taper off (or society might cease to function!). But that doesn't mean that you can't continue to have terrific sex.

A TALE OF TWO VAGINAS

ANNIE, AN OLD FRIEND, OPENED UP to me that she and her husband of eighteen years were going through a sexual renaissance after a long and sometimes tense drought. Their sex life dropped off after they had kids. When she hit perimenopause she also started to experience vaginal dryness that made sex uncomfortable and even upsetting, but she didn't consider speaking with her doctor or using a lubricant—she thought that was just the way it was going to be. She resorted to giving her husband the occasional blow job, which triggered wrought feelings of being pushed into having sex as a much younger woman. Out of fear she was going to "lead him on," she stopped being cuddly and warm at all. Meanwhile, her husband, who is someone who craves physical expressions of love, felt rejected and resentful. And neither of them was talking about it. The coldness began to pervade their entire relationship.

Couples therapy might have helped them figure all of this out, but instead it was an argument. After a gale-force falling out over something at the level of dishwasher-loading feng shui, they got real. She admitted that sex had started to be painful and emotionally loaded; he reassured her that the main thing he needed was physical closeness. This was an opportunity to reboot. The next date night started with cocktails and a trip to a woman-friendly sex shop and ended with lube, a vibrator, light restraints, and multiple orgasms.

Sex therapist Esther Perel's brilliant book *Mating in Captivity* addresses the paradox of wanting both adventure and security in monogamous relationships, and she nails it just right when she says, "When there is nothing left to hide, there is nothing left to seek." Unfortunately, there's no easy solution to this conundrum; everything's a trade-off. But she says, and I agree, that communication, as scary as it can be, is essential, just as Annie and her husband ultimately realized.

It's been drilled into most of us (and rightly so) not to have sex when we aren't feeling it. This is important advice for a twenty-year-old but doesn't always benefit a woman in a safe, mature, long-term relationship. The simplest step to switch on your sexual drive is to reach out to your partner, even when you aren't feeling amorous. According to Ian Kerner, PhD, therapist and author of the bestseller *She Comes First,* "People often have this funny idea that sex has to begin with desire, but science has shown the opposite." He continues, "Especially for women, arousal often leads to desire." Kerner adds that while men can experience spontaneous arousal (that would be, in layman's terms, an erection popping up out of nowhere), women experience responsive desire, which requires more of a context (think oily massage, reading an erotic novel, lying together on the beach). He suggests that couples in a sexual rut "put their bodies in motion and see if that leads to desire." One advantage of sharing a bed with the same person for years is that if it doesn't work today, you can always try again tomorrow.

UNFAITHFULLY YOURS

NO ONE KNOWS WHAT GOES ON inside a marriage except for the two people in it, and by the time you've hit our age, you've very likely seen it all, if not in your own relationship, then in those of the people around you. As one of my girlfriends recently put it, "I've been the cheater, and I've been cheated on. I've tried all the positions."

We're raised to think that adultery would be the death knell for every relationship, and it often is, but not always. As Esther Perel says, "Not every infidelity is a symptom of a problem in a relationship. Sometimes it has to do with other longings that are much more existential. Sometimes you go elsewhere not because you are not liking the one you are with; you are not liking the person you have become." Never is this more true, perhaps, than in our later years, when who we have become is looking more and more like the last stop on the train.

As one of the Woolfers opined,

> Honestly, I think we have all been cheated on and have cheated on in some way...it's the level of violation, the associated meaning that matters...couples don't end relationships because of an affair, emotional or physical, we have affairs because we are unhappy and dissatisfied. We are standing up and saying, I did this because I was unhappy. It doesn't preclude the opportunity for the couple to move forward, or that the love they feel for one another can't prevail, but that takes honesty with ourselves and with each other.

There's no easy answer on this front. Monogamy is boring some-times, but it's also romantic (he's mine, I'm his). Infidelity is exciting (God, the thought of a new person craving me, touching me), but it's also exhausting (the lies, the maneuvering) and generally a sign of real inner distress, and who wants that? If what you are really after is blowing up your life, having an affair is very effective but usually comes with significant collateral damage. I never feel judgment about other people's affairs. Having been there myself, I just feel sad for the parties involved.

OPEN MARRIAGES

AS I UNDERSTAND IT, COMMON WISDOM on open marriages is that, as appealing as they sometimes sound (how I wouldn't kill for two husbands, some days), they don't work. I'm an incredibly jealous person, and I'd be completely torn apart if I was asked to tolerate my husband romancing another woman, not to mention him penetrating her body. That's way more than I could ever han-dle, even though there's admittedly a level of sexiness about it—the notion of seeing him in that way again, as a seducer, as a pure object of desire and not the guy who farts in bed sometimes—that can turn me on for a hot second. But for me, it's not worth the trade-off.

There are people who do it and swear by it. Here's a story from a girlfriend:

I'm nineteen years into a marriage with two kids (eight and twelve) and am openly seeing someone else. My husband knows when I see this man, and when I spend the night with him we make up a lie to the kids about where I am. At this time, he has no interest in pursuing another relationship. In couples counseling he said he felt relieved that I'm involved with someone else—that he knows he doesn't meet my emotional or physical needs himself, and hasn't for years (we have sex maybe twice a year and we sleep in separate bedrooms). All my husband wants, I think, is to keep our family together so he can be with the kids full-time, rather than divorcing. And divorce is so expensive—we're both hypereducated, with careers, but the cost of maintaining two separate homes is too overwhelming at the moment. But, I do find it difficult to be in two relationships at the same time, even though only one of them is intimate. It is psychically draining somehow. For the time being it helps with my financial stability and the stability of the kids' lives.

Another friend, a divorced writer in her midfifties, fell hard last year for a fellow writer, a guy who was in an open marriage of more than two decades. The connection was intense on all levels, mostly sexually and intellectually, and at first she liked the heat of being the "allowed" mistress. But six months later, after really falling in love, being perpetually consigned to the number two slot got to be too painful, and she had to end it. It broke her heart.

I doubt you're just learning now that love is complicated and there are no easy answers. The sad truth of the matter is that from what I see and hear, it never gets any easier.

FEMALE EJACULATION AND THE ELUSIVE G-SPOT

I long ago gave up on finding my G-spot, really just out of laziness and also because I've been pretty happy with my regular orgasms. But lately, a lot of my fifty-plus girlfriends are boasting about this crazy "squirting" thing they can suddenly do. And yes, everyone hates that word, and yet, somehow, it persists.

It's a real phenomenon, I swear, even though I've not yet experienced it. Even Aristotle made mention of female ejaculation. In the Tantric religion, female ejaculate is referred to as *amrita*, which translates to "the nectar of the Gods." Galen of Pergamon once wrote that female ejaculate "manifestly flows from women as they experience the greatest pleasure in coitus."

Let's get clear on our terms and the details:

- The G-spot, or the female prostate, is an erogenous zone tucked inside the vagina. The ejaculate, however, is expelled from the urethra. For this reason, women often worry that the fluid they've ejected in passion is pee, and nothing takes the sexy out of sex quite like being accused of peeing on someone—for most people, anyway. It's not pee, in that it doesn't come from the bladder, but it does indeed share some of the same chemical components of urine—namely, urea and creatinine—but I suggest we don't get too technical and enjoy the ride.

- It's apparently a different kind of orgasm (everyone I talk to says not better, though, just different) that involves female ejaculate, a gushing of fluid.
- Every woman is capable of experiencing ejaculation and supposedly we can all learn how to make this happen. There are toys and books on the subject, if you're looking for a new adventure.

EVE: As the author of *The Goddess Orgasm* I can say, professionally, that many, many women can squirt. And most of them are stunned, if not embarrassed, the first time it happens. It's really a wonderful thing and don't be afraid of it. But also if it's never happened to you, don't lose sleep over it.

DELIA: The first time it happened to me I was sniffing the bed too! It's so crazy!! My lover said I was gushing; I was sure it was urine. But it's clear and scent-free. I agree the orgasms are not necessarily better. It's the same but with an added extraordinary wet release. I love it. It started for me after menopause. People say you can learn it, and you probably can, but for me it just started happening like I grew a G-spot overnight.

MARYANNE: A friend of mine here in Buenos Aires also recently started "squirting" at fifty-five. Very much looking forward.

ELISA: I got it in menopause too and thought of it as gushing or slushing or rushing, like rushing waters (marginally better than "squirting"). Not a more intense orgasm—it's as if the release dampens it—but great!

WAIT, WHICH WAY DO I SWIPE?

*Sex is one of the three best things out there, and
I don't even know what the other two are.*
—HELEN GURLEY BROWN

THERE ARE SO MANY THINGS you don't want to hear on a first date. I surveyed a bunch of women and came up with a brief list of four word stunners that should make you run in the other direction:

"Can my mom come?"

"It doesn't itch much."

"I love Michael Bolton."

"I hate my mother."

"Feminists are so angry."

"I'm in a cult."

"You think too much."

"My ex is insane."

"I hate pushy women."

"You are ordering that?"

"Why don't you smile?"

The answer to the last question would be, "Because I'm sitting across the table from an asshole like you." But I digress.

What's it like to be out there single, dating, and having sex as we slide into middle age and beyond? I've done it all. I had a sixteen-year marriage that ended when I was thirty-seven, spent eight years dating, and remarried at forty-five. And like you, I'm sure, I have many single friends. It's hard to pin down an exact number of women over forty who are dating (as opposed to in a long-term relationship but not married or simply not interested) but based on the number of women in the online dating pool, it's at least 30 million.

A word on setups: In this age of online dating, everyone so wishes they could meet a partner "the old-fashioned way," either randomly at a party (that is, I admit, how I wound up meeting hubby number two) or from a setup. I found setups, however, to be oddly misleading. Because a setup is generally a mutual friend, the person always *seems* right for you (a known quantity, same class/educational background, vetted), so I found I was more likely to jump right in. In fact, I confess I slept with every single man my friends set me up with during my postdivorce dating years. But they weren't the right guys for me. Connection and chemistry are so mysterious, and who we think is right for us is often not who really stirs our loins, so to speak. That said, I'm a fan of online dating, as difficult as it can be. It gets you out there, it's good practice, and there's a shitload of variety.

For me, the hardest part about online dating was all the rejection (again, the setups are easier that way, but so much less surprising). I have four kids and am half-black, so I think immediately my online profile must have scared certain men off. Lying about your age is one thing (which I never did, but I totally understand why some do), but erasing my children just plain seems like bad karma, and I never went there. So you're out there, exposed for the world to see, on the Internet looking for love. There are so many ways to go—do you respond to every seemingly inappropriate guy who approaches you? Ignore everyone but the ones who seem perfect? Do you "wink" at guys or only wait 'til they approach you? Everyone figures out their own rules, but here were mine:

NINA'S INTERNET DATING RULES

1. Unless you're quite confident you're going to like the dude, don't agree to drinks or dinner. Drinking will make you more likely to sleep with someone you don't really want to sleep with. Start with coffee, nice and sober.

2. Don't waste time with too much emailing or too many phone calls beforehand. Just meet for coffee. You can actually fall in love with someone over the phone and then when you meet them in person feel *zero* chemistry. This has happened to me and it's *very* hard to extricate yourself, trust me.

3. If you wink at or write to or swipe someone and they ignore you, *try, try, try* to not take it personally. You have no idea what's going on in that person's life. He may be involved with two other people; he may have a particular hang-up about your hair color; he may be out of the country. You simply won't know, and this guy doesn't know you from Eve, so it's not personal. He's just not the one.

4. You may be a more generous person than me, but I say don't respond to all the completely uninteresting people who message you. It's a huge time suck and you wind up arguing with strangers about why you don't want to go out with them. I felt like the better tactic was to ignore. For follow-ups on dates that you don't want to pursue, come up with a standard one- or two-liner that fits all occasions, something like "Dear so-and-so, you are a great guy, but I don't feel we were a match. Good luck to you."

5. Keep your profile up even when you are discouraged. You can take breaks from how intensely you engage with the sites, but keep your profile up. It's a numbers game, and an evergreen one. There's always another guy out there hitting the market (getting divorced, widowed, ready to date) and you just never know when a really intriguing person is going to send you a sweet note… and he will, I promise.

Unfortunately, even when Mr. (or Ms.) Seemingly Almost Perfect does come calling, it might not be smooth sailing. We're all older now, we come with our issues—mountains of emotional baggage, physical imperfections—and we're stuck in our ways.

Since I have been married again for a few years and out of the singles game, I invited two women who are actively dating for tea and a candid conversation. Cathy, forty-nine, is a film executive and has never been married. Being sexual has always been a big part of her identity. She's tall, blond, outspoken, and stylish, and people often compare her to Samantha on *Sex and the City* (which bugs the hell out of her because she doesn't want to be seen as a cliché or type.) Her best friend, Rachel, fifty, is an artist, was married for a few years, and now has two teenage kids. Aside from the usual travails of online dating, what stuck out for me most during our talk was how, by their late forties and early fifties, it was the men who felt especially self-conscious and decrepit.

"Most of the time sex starts out badly," said Cathy. "Men often can't get it up the first time because of the usual erectile issues of aging, but also because they are insecure about their bodies (being overweight, their sagging gut, et cetera), which has a psychological effect on their penises."

Rachel added, "There's also a lot of insecurity about their existential selves—mortality to deal with, meaning-of-life stuff…"

Every expert I spoke with mentioned that as much as women worry about being sexy after forty, one of the big reasons "vanilla" sex isn't working is because of male dysfunction. In contrast to the way mature men and women are portrayed in the media (i.e., studly vs. withered), in real life, the opposite is often true. I feel compassion for men in this situation, but reminding oneself of this can be a revelation.

As with long relationships and potentially drooping dicks, Cathy said that ED drugs are a sensitive but necessary topic to broach. "Yes, you have to persist. It's fine if you really like them, but if I don't, I find myself trying to think up ways to get them out of my bed ASAP. If you want a relationship to work, suggest some Viagra. But I say, 'Because it makes sex more fun,' which allows them to save face."

"Right," Rachel said, laughing. "More, 'Let's have kinky time with our sex organs pumped up with blood like a couple of bonobos,' than, 'Can you please take some Viagra so your cock stops resembling a used tea bag?'"

Both women said that body confidence is a turn-on even if their dates aren't as smooth, taut, and muscled as they once were. (Note to women: men feel the same way.) Cathy recently reconnected with a boyfriend, Jonathan, from her college days. "His body was less than perfect, but he strode around my apartment naked and that was a turn-on."

A notable upside to dating and shagging an older guy is that they, like we, have probably picked up a few tricks along the way. I definitely have found this to be the case. Surprise, surprise, lots of men are good at sex! "Jonathan had learned so much since we were together in college," she said. "He knew exactly how to get me off while having sex—using his fingers on my clitoris—so I actually had an orgasm during penetration, which is rare for me."

Rachel said that it could be "hideous" to get naked for the first time after "covering up for a few years," and she dreaded that moment when you have to get up and walk to the bathroom, but she agreed that sex for her was better at this age because she was far more honest and less inhibited.

Then there's the entertainment factor. Online dating at our age can be a bonding experience with your girlfriends: even in a city as large as New York, the over-forty or over-fifty dating pool online is just not that big, and if you do it for long enough, you may find some overlap. I was having drinks with two friends who were talking about their forays on OkCupid. One described a guy she had been seeing for a couple of weeks. The other suddenly asked, "Does he write crime fiction? Wear wire-rimmed glasses? Really into eating pussy?" Check. Check. Check. "Ah, yes. The Novelist." Things got a little quiet and awkward; it kind of felt like they were one degree away from cheating—or being in a threesome.

There's no easy answer here. Relationships are hard and dating is hard. And they can also both be lots of fun. There's nothing like the thrill of meeting someone new and feeling that intensity of emotion in the pit of your stomach, and there are Sunday mornings in bed with my husband where I feel like I've hit the jackpot in love. But there are also fights that we revisit way too often, and my single girlfriends call me sobbing when guy X or Y turns out to be a huge disappointment. Life is a struggle. At our age, though, after speaking with so many women, my advice is that you should at least be prepared for some ED issues and also try to be clear about your own sexual and intimacy needs. What are the traits you are looking for in a partner? Then cut that list in half, take some cute selfies, and get yourself on Tinder or Bumble, because life is short and we all want connection.

DIM ALL THE LIGHTS: THE UNFUCKABILITY FACTOR

HOW DO WE FEEL ABOUT becoming less visible, or as Amy Schumer and Tiny Fey put it, "unfuckable"? Is there a middle-aged woman alive who has not seen their sheer genius "Last Fuckable

Day" video? If you've somehow missed, it, I implore you to put this book down for a moment and go straight to YouTube.

Now that you're back, let's talk about not feeling desirable. A couple of years ago, *Humans of New York* featured a beautiful older woman who said, "The world doesn't respond to me like it used to." She went on to discuss the difficult period of transition when she suddenly felt she had become less "visible" and the way people treated her seemed to have changed. She realized then how many social transactions she experienced over her lifetime were based on her beauty and youth. It was upsetting, but eventually she said, "There's a certain grace to letting go of the need for attention."

I'm all over the map on this. Yes, at times I fret that nobody would want me anymore: my body is too slack, I'm past my prime, I'm faded. Often the biggest obstacles are the voices in our own heads. For starters, we don't become unfuckable to those who love us. Conventional wisdom says that men feel pretty lucky to get sexual attention when they get it, and if you've made him come hundreds of times, he probably still likes it when you do it again. And for me, out in the world, I am starting to enjoy a power in being viewed less as an object of physical beauty and more for who I am. To be truly seen. Spun that way, we actually become *more* visible with age. Do we really want to be recognized primarily for our desirability? What is that kind of attention really worth? It's nice to attract a partner, certainly, but beyond that? Worth considering: lose the "wrong" kind of visibility and discover a whole other level of potential within ourselves? I can be happy with that trade.

On the whole, I'm happier with my sex life now than I've been at any other time in my life to date. I orgasm easily, I'm not shy about asking for what I want, I like to fantasize, and I'm psyched to climb into bed with my partner, even if we both may have some inevitable age-related dysfunction from time to time. Expert Levkoff said to me, "We have power, we're in a more secure stage of our lives; there can be an amazing sense of freedom in our bodies and a devil-may-care attitude about sex." Of all the draggy parts of getting old, I'm not finding sex to be one of them. I encourage you to enjoy your hard-earned self-knowledge and cut loose in the sack. You aren't twenty-five—yay!—you don't have to deal with the bullshit expectations and hang-ups that younger women struggle with. And remember, a little lube goes a long way.

CHAPTER THREE

(BODIES)

IS EVERYTHING SAGGING OR IS IT JUST ME?

Stop whining about getting old. It's a privilege.
—AMY POEHLER

MY NO-DENIAL MOMENT ABOUT MY declining body came when I was forty-five. I'm sure there had been plenty of times before this when I started noticing a general collapse (I confess I started using Botox at thirty-eight, for example, but more on that later), but the real "holy crap, this is only going in one direction" moment happened at our country's infamous Mall of America. I was traveling with my eldest daughter, then twenty-one, to visit my son, her brother, at school. We flew into the Minneapolis airport and had some time to kill, so we decided to check out the ginormous shopping emporium less than a mile away.

We found ourselves in Madewell, trying on jeans. We were both a size six, give or take. This seemed promising to me. She was no longer a gangly fourteen-year-old, and I was not a more matronly size fourteen. I was proud of how beautiful my daughter looked, and also so glad to see what appeared to me a completely relaxed state about her size and what fit how. I was handing her sizes and styles over the door of the changing room, as mothers do, and then taking some of her leftovers and trying them on myself. This all felt like great fun, until we both happened to be inside the changing room at the same time, trying on the same size and style, a simple black denim, waist twenty-eight. The pants were a little too big on my daughter and a little too snug on me. Her body looked firm and adorable, and my gut was hanging over the waist of my jeans. Looking in the mirror, the pants looked eh (at best) on me and stunning on her.

As bright as day, I suddenly realized that no matter what size or weight I am, my body has changed—and will keep changing. An ineffable awareness came upon me that no matter how hard I exercise or diet or what clothes I wear, I am no longer a young woman. This is particularly hard to avoid noticing when standing naked in a small mirrored space with a genuinely young woman right next to you. And if that young woman is your daughter, there's both a beautiful quality (the pride, the turning over of the generations) and a horrifying one (I created her and now I'm over the hill and useless) to this particular epiphany.

It's no coincidence that I was in the throes of perimenopause during this experience. As we enter our forties and estrogen production begins to wane, most of us will notice a shape-shifting from the typical hourglass shape to, let's say, a more solid rectangle, or even a shot-glass sort of shape, if you will. When we were younger, all that estrogen coursing through our supple systems was directing fat deposits onto our hips, thighs, and asses, which are the repositories of calories used for breast-feeding. Now that our feeding capability is no longer an issue, our fat preferentially deposits in a more male-like pattern, around and inside our abdomens. This is why when I was in that dressing room with my daughter, I was suddenly seeing strange bulges where she had none. This observation was not my hyperactive imagination. The other day my friend Sara said, "In the last year, my body seems to be changing at warp speed, especially my fat distribution." She's right.

In addition to our ever-altering contours, as we age our bodies start going through countless internal changes and some (hopefully not too many) indignities. The question is, how do we deal with all this with grace and not too much bitterness and self-criticism?

Women's health guru Christiane Northrup, MD, is renowned for her truly brilliant books on women's health and spiritual well-being. I trust her medical advice and have often found myself googling her expert opinion. Dr. Northrup is particularly known for her visionary approach to wellness and self-love, which includes the unity of mind, body, emotions, and spirit. I bring her up here because in theory, I think her exhortation should be ours: "Embrace your ageless goddess!" Yes! She says in her most famous tome, *Women's Bodies, Women's Wisdom*, "Thoughts are an important part of your inner wisdom and they are very powerful. A thought held long enough and repeated often enough becomes a belief. A belief then becomes your biology." Hallelujah…Well, maybe.

On the one hand I totally want to celebrate my beauty and power and know myself in a new and deeper way and believe that my health and wellness are in my control. On the other hand, I feel like that's an awful lot of pressure. Can't I sometimes feel sorry for myself? Is it really my own fault if I get arthritis? I don't think so…

We can allow room for both things to be true: if you have embraced your ageless inner queen and couldn't care less about your muffin top or back fat, then right on, sister! But if you're ambivalent and sometimes feel a tad body dysmorphic, I'm here to tell you that you are not alone. Research out of Stanford University finds that, as during puberty, at this stage of life women are at a higher risk for developing eating disorders (although the numbers are thankfully lower than when we were teens). A 2012 study in the *International Journal of Eating Disorders* found that 13 percent of women over fifty exhibit some related symptoms such as binge eating and/or purging, extreme exercising, or excessive dieting. Moreover, 60 percent say that their body dissatisfaction or preoccupation with weight negatively impacts their lives, and 70 percent report that they are bothered by their weight. These numbers surprised me when I first read them, but they shouldn't have. Of course our culture's infatuation with youth, beauty, and thinness dovetails with the reality of changing bodies (plus...you guessed it...hormones!) in a way that makes some women feel like crap on a daily basis.

An anonymous post in the group really brought to life the many paradoxes inherent in how we feel about our changing bodies and lives:

> I mourn how my aging face and body has changed the way my husband responds to me. I notice that he gets a spring in his step around a young beauty and sort of trips all over himself in her presence. I am not a careerist, my kids are grown and doing well I may add, but what am I? I am way too old to be a trophy wife, not much homemaking left to do. I'm writing a book and volunteering but feel invisible and somewhat

boring. When we are in the bloom of youth, the men in our lives may not give a hoot about our earning potential, especially if we are beautiful. We are their sex objects, their pride, their partners and the mothers of their (born or unborn) children. But as we age, and perhaps get gray, saggy, fat, or worse—sick—they are less doting, more critical. They revere us, but there is a change. I've noticed this across the board among my friends. They question our maintenance (your hair costs that much! why do you need new shoes?). It can be a sad state of affairs. And perhaps this is why some of us fight aging so aggressively, starving ourselves, exercising like mad, spending on anti-aging creams and cures. And yet though he still makes love to us, we also catch him admiring the waitress's firmer, perkier ass. So, what I'm asking for is a rethink. We must reinvent ourselves. We are not cute. We are not fertile. We are smart, capable people who can still achieve in the world. We cannot age out, nor give up, or else we will just stay in our bathrobes all day. We must take ourselves seriously. Not chase youth or feel ashamed, but support each other and forge ahead.

Understandably, this struck a chord, and responses rolled in:

JESSICA: Agreed. Though you couldn't pay me enough money to go back to the days when I had a perkier ass... I am 1000% stronger and more interesting now!

ESTELLE: Yes, but one thing I finally learned upon turning 40 is this—we no longer have to give a fuck. This is the time to dye, to nip, to tuck, to strut, to run, to eat, to say what is on your mind, to try new things, to scare yourself, to fail and realize—hell yeah there is time to try again—or not—IT'S YOUR CALL. Let him stare at that waitress's ass, let him hop skip and step at a young thing, but let me tell you, sexy isn't that ass, it's you being you—ALL you—without compromise, without the fear of what others will think. Spend money on your hair, buy the shoes, drink the wine—we think you're sexy and worth it just the way you are.

SHARON: We decide how to value ourselves, and what is beautiful, really. If we let society (and those who are enslaved to its fluctuating ideas of beauty and worth) decide, we will always be chasing after something that eludes us. And if we feel beautiful in our vitality, focus, kindness, wisdom, creativity, etc., others are more likely to respond to that.

LISA: It's unfortunate how much looks and youth (especially in women) are valued in our society and how insidious and pervasive the message is that these qualities are so important. I have always worked as a professional and am relatively proud of my career achievements so I don't struggle too much in that area of my life, but I can totally relate to feeling more "invisible" as I age. I know youth and beauty are fleeting (and frankly I never felt particularly attractive in my younger years...) but nonetheless I am now acutely aware of a shift in the way I am perceived. I know it shouldn't matter and doesn't matter to the people who I am closest to, but nonetheless I notice it. I am hoping that as I age I will start to get used to it more, and I will stop noticing it.

ROBIN: It's true that our youth-obsessed culture works against the aging physique. And it seems worse for women, but why? I'm not too psyched about my husband's body either and I flirt like crazy and get psyched when a younger dude gives me attention. So, it's not strictly a male disposition. Aging sucks! If you can't find some other way of relating to your spouse, then maybe it's time to move on?

MADELINE: There really is the possibility of more and better. We're mostly, with luck and care, healthier than "old ladies" were in earlier times; some of us have been lucky enough to integrate yoga or long walks or biking or the gym and our butts are mighty nice, especially in skinnies or Lulu's. Staying out of the sun or using sunblock has helped our skin so much and we're still curious, feisty, whimsical, sexual, and vain (sorry, but I think some amount of vanity is fab) and know how to eat well. You might, thanks to all of the above, have a better sex life than you did with child raising and work when you really, really just wanted to sleep. I remain hopeful.

What stunning responses, and so full of love, right? Which does sort of bring us back to Christiane Northrup. We need to be gentle with ourselves, and also courageous. I *do* care about how I look and I *am* willing to put some effort into it. I'm not going to lie about my vanity or cover up my occasional unhappiness with my appearance. But I'm much more focused on being healthy and strong and vital for as long as possible, and being a decent role model for my daughters in this regard. Not saying the self-critical stuff aloud ad nauseam is probably healthy for my own self-image anyway. Wrestling with all of this and being open about it is the way I cope. So this is not a chapter about self-hatred (the endlessly fine line) but rather a "let's be honest about the ignominies of physically aging, and both see what little we can do about it *and* support one another and love ourselves anyway." Who's game?

Note: the kicker with this thread about our physically aging bodies was that Anonymous followed up a few weeks later letting us all know that our conversation inspired her to speak to her husband honestly, and the result has been dates and love notes and adoration. He's afraid of losing her! A win-win all around.

YOU ARE WHAT YOU EAT. REALLY.

THERE ARE A MILLION DIET and exercise books out there, and I may not say anything you haven't heard before. What works for me might not work at all for you. For me, the "no white food" rule is a good one. No dairy, no sugar, no bread. I try to eat tons of fresh fruits and vegetables every day, limit red meat in favor of chicken and fish, don't drink coffee, try (endlessly try) to limit my alcohol consumption. I believe in beans, even though my personal favorite diet, the Whole30, does not, but I do try to limit my grains as that eating plan recommends, because no matter how healthy quinoa and farro may be, they make me feel bloated. Listen to your body.

Karen Tayeh, registered dietician nutritionist (and Woolfer!), explained to me what most of us probably intuitively know: even if you are eating as healthfully and exercising the same amount as you always did, it's likely you'll lose muscle mass and gain weight as you get older. "If everything is the status quo, you might not be able to maintain, let alone lose weight," she said. "To slow the process, you'll need to ramp up your exercise, and eat cleaner and cleaner." If you haven't been strength training to build muscle, now is the time to start.

Tayeh suggests eating lean proteins (such as salmon, chicken without skin, beans, and tofu), which help fuel muscle repair. She also recommends being picky about the amount and type of carbs you consume. As your cells are aging, they aren't as efficient at getting glucose out of your bloodstream. Excess glucose is converted to fat, or worse, can lead to diabetes. Glucose comes from *any* carb, from brown rice to kale to chocolate chip cookies (and wine!). (See the next section, "Booze," for more on alcohol.) "You still need energy from glucose as well as the nutrients that come from whole grains, fruits, and vegetables, so focus on cutting back on the empty carbs. Be mindful about treats but don't completely deprive yourself, as that can backfire." Tayeh is a fan of good fats like avocado, olive oil, nuts, and seeds eaten in moderation. She explains that one benefit of these fats is they help build aging cell walls and keep your hair, nails, and skin looking healthy. Staying hydrated is also key. Another must is eating antioxidant-rich foods. Antioxidants scavenge the free radicals that can damage cells and lead to diseases like cancer, heart disease, and Alzheimer's. Excellent and easy-to-find sources are dark grapes, blueberries, broccoli, and kidney beans. The idea of eating super-clean can feel really tedious, but understanding the benefits is motivating. It's also one of the few factors truly under our control.

BOOZE: THE PROS AND MOSTLY CONS

SPOILER ALERT: YOU MAY WANT to skip this section. I certainly will not enjoy writing it. I love wine, and now that wine gives me insomnia and hot flashes (distilled spirits, particularly vodka and tequila, which are gluten- and sugar-free, seem to be the friendliest tipple for this middle-aged lady), I've discovered a love of *reposado* tequila mixed with fresh lime juice, shaken with lots of ice, and served in a chilled martini glass. To me, this is menopausal nirvana after a hard day. No cloying sweetness, elegant, delicious. That said, here goes:

Anything more than very light alcohol consumption is quite simply very bad for us, pretty much across the board. Whatever minute gains there may be in reducing risk of heart disease, dementia, diabetes, and obesity (all with "moderate" drinking, i.e., no more than seven drinks per week and never more than three drinks on any single day), the fact is *any* amount of alcohol increases the risk of breast cancer and cancer in general. Women who drink two to five drinks a day have about one and a half times the risk of nondrinkers. The National Institute on Alcohol and Alcohol Abuse (NIAAA) warns that women who drink heavily are more vulnerable to alcohol-related brain, heart, and liver disease than their male counterparts. Drinking also seems to trigger and worsen hot flashes for some women, although I'm making that claim purely based on anecdotal research (every woman I know over forty, that is).

Once you start drinking heavily (anything more than moderate), it's a train wreck. The most recent study I could get my hands on while writing this book (from May 2017 by the American Institute for Cancer Research) reports that just one drink a day increases the risk of breast cancer for postmenopausal women by 9 percent.

According to the NIAAA, alcohol has the following effects on your health:

- It increases the risk of cardiovascular disease. Among heavy drinkers, women are more susceptible to alcohol-related heart disease than men.

- It increases the risk of central obesity—the apple shape that is a big risk for cardiovascular disease.

- It increases the risk of irreversible osteoporosis.

- It increases the risk for fractures.

- It increases the risk of developing type 2 diabetes.

- It is a depressant, and menopausal women are already especially vulnerable to depression, so drinking can just make that worse.

NINA'S VIRGINIA WOOLF COCKTAIL

That's the bad news. If you have the very occasional cocktail, you'll thank me for this, the good news. It's delicious and elegant—the mature woman's cosmo!—and it's literally the only thing I drink these days. It won't keep you up at night or give you headaches (as long as you stick to just one; after that I can't make any promises) or make you feel like you just ate three chocolate croissants.

Ingredients:
¼ cup tequila
½ cup fresh, unsweetened lime juice

Shake the tequila and lime juice in a chilled shaker with lots of ice, pour to the rim of a classic martini glass, and present with a lime twist. Cheers!

SUGAR IS THE ENEMY

SUGAR IS REALLY, REALLY BAD for us, and I find as I get older that I can't tolerate it. Any sugar I eat, I feel. I'm instantly bloated, sleep badly, and notice it in my skin, which gets duller and drier, sort of on the way to sandpaper territory.

Added sugar (table sugar, the high-fructose corn syrup found in soda, other processed sweeteners, and, yes, even honey and maple syrup) may be particularly bad for the perimenopausal woman because of (yes, again) our fluctuating hormones, but here's the skinny on why it's just plain bad for everyone, according to the nutrition experts at the website Authority Nutrition:

- It contains no essential nutrients.

- Fructose (found in added sugar, fruit, and some vegetables) doesn't have the same kind of effect on feeling full as glucose (grains, legumes, etc.); it makes us eat more.

- Large amounts of fructose can raise triglycerides; small, dense LDL; oxidized LDL; blood glucose and insulin levels; and can increase abdominal obesity, all major risk factors for heart disease.

- It's bad for your teeth because it feeds the harmful bacteria in the mouth.

■ Fructose can be processed only by the liver, so it burdens the liver and can lead to nonalcoholic liver disease.

■ It causes insulin resistance, which can lead to diabetes.

■ It causes inflammation, which can lead to cancer.

■ Researchers now understand that insulin resistance is a powerful force in the development of Alzheimer's disease.

■ It causes dopamine release, so it's addictive.

Not all carbs are equal, even ones that contain fructose. Compare a piece of fruit to a candy bar. The fruit is fiber-rich, which makes you feel full and slows the absorption of sugar, and is loaded with vitamins and antioxidants, while the candy bar is essentially nutritional garbage. You can get much more technical and compare a certain food's glycemic index (how much "sugar" it contains) to its glycemic load (how quickly it raises your blood sugar levels), but suffice it to say you probably already know the difference between a carrot and a doughnut.

All that said, I suggest playing with your intake. Try cutting out all added sugars for a week or two—heaps of white sugar in your iced coffee and silly sweet cocktails are the easiest to dump—and I pretty much guarantee you'll feel better. At the very least, I'd wager that you'll notice better sleep and steadier energy levels.

ROW, ROW, ROW, YOUR BELLY BLOAT

TUMMY BLOATING IS ALSO VERY common for women our age. While it's important to rule out a more serious medical condition (ovarian cancer, anyone? Crohn's disease?), it's thought to be caused by the ever-present and annoying hormonal fluctuations. One of the many roles estrogen plays in our bodies is in the maintenance of water and bile. As the estrogen levels start to shift, our bodies tend to store more water, making us feel (and look) bloated. In addition, the amount of bile we produce begins to change, so the way we digest fats does too, which sadly leads to more gas being produced in the digestive system. Unfortunately, many of the foods that are recommended to maintain a healthy BMI, reduce perimenopause symptoms, and prevent bone loss—high-fiber grains and vegetables, soy, milk products—also produce gas. So, yes, we fart more, apparently as much as 30 to 60 percent more than when we were younger. How lovely.

LAURIE: Egads—a sudden preponderance to bloat? No diet changes, but pregnancy-size bloating. Aside from sticking a pin in my belly, any suggestions?

I totally related to this post. When my perimenopause went into full gear, I was bloating like crazy and the worst were my breasts— they felt like my milk was coming in. The answer for me was entirely related to dietary changes; when I gave up all alcohol, gluten, dairy, and sugar (an extreme move, I know, and not sustainable), the bloating disappeared and my breasts felt normal again. It's very common.

NANCY: I googled this over the weekend! I'm in the same b(l)oat.

SUSAN: The bloating and big boobs have been the biggest surprise to me. Agree that diet changes seem to make a difference. It's hard for me to stick to all the time but even a few days of limiting sugar and alcohol feels like it makes a difference. I also rotate lactose-free milk into coffee/tea as much as possible.

CARLA: This is a common side effect of hormonal changes. Usually, the culprits are onion, garlic (sorry), but I found that eliminating gluten from my diet also helped. Also, sugar substitutes are known irritants, and they all should be eliminated.

HILLARY: I had bloating and extreme breast tenderness (particularly the latter) even before (these years), and when I quit Diet Coke—boom, COMPLETELY gone. DC was my caffeine source, and for years when I would mention the breast tenderness to the OB/GYN, I was told it could be a factor.

Basically it's not rocket science: change your eating habits. For you it might mean cutting out dairy, for me it may be sugar, but the bottom line is, if you're bloating, your body is reacting to something that isn't working for you anymore. Figure out what it is with an elimination diet (one week no milk, the next no gluten, until you a work through potential triggers), and you'll feel and look better. Also, more of the obvious: drink lots of water and exercise more, both of which are beneficial in so many ways—brighter skin, lubricated joints, mood boost, and so on.

CONSTIPATION, GAS, REFLUX...OH JOY

My friend Dr. Jenny Breznay, a gerontologist and family medicine expert, says that this trio "may be the final frontier" of what's not discussed enough with aging. "Nothing makes you feel more like your grandmother," and yet these gastro issues all become increasingly common as we age. Jenny explains it like this: our guts are sort of like our brains, and both organs start to enervate, or slow down, as we get older. If we're not moving as much as we used to, that will make us sluggish on the inside as well. Also, we're just plain drier all over, inside and out, and the dehydration stops us up. Lastly, if we're taking any medications, which we're more likely to be doing now, they often affect bowel transmitters, and that will cause problems. So: move, hydrate, and be aware of side effects of the meds!

THE FOUR HORSEMEN (BAT WINGS, BACK FAT, MUFFIN TOP, PAUNCH)

DO ALL MY BODY EPIPHANIES take place in dressing rooms? A few months ago I was in a fabulous New York City discount fashion emporium (Century 21) trying on drastically reduced spring dresses from Marni and Missoni, when all of a sudden I caught a horrifying glimpse of chicken skin under my arms. It was unmistakable. Until that moment I actually thought my arms were doing pretty well. I lift weights so they're toned, and I have triceps muscles you can sort of see if you squint and the lighting is just so. My biceps are not embarrassing. But the truth is, no matter what I do, I'm getting older and my skin is going to start hanging off my body! This is totally unavoidable. All of us, depending on our various genetic makeups and lifestyles, will start to develop at least one of the above-referenced four horsemen—back fat, muffin top, paunch, and bat wings. You could starve yourself (don't) and exercise hard, and maybe you would put them off for a few years, but they are coming for you. Sorry!

To this point, I was heartened and delighted with this post in the group:

> ***MARTIA:*** The biggest surprise while cleaning out my closet today was how many perfectly good clothes were hidden in the back—and that I had stopped even seeing—because they were waiting for me to "lose a few pounds so I can wear them again." And the issue was very specific: those clothes showed my increasing muffin top. Guess what? If I stop comparing myself to the "perfect" body, I can wear all those clothes NOW!! I feel liberated!
> Embrace the MUFFIN TOP!
> I'm pulling those clothes to the front of the closet. And I promise to wear them—no, not just to wear them

but to PRANCE around town in them! I'm LOLing with relief and letting go. What did I think would happen if I had worn those clothes the last couple years and let my muffin top show? That people would notice? (Some would, some wouldn't.) That people would be mean to me or reject me or think less of me? (They wouldn't.) It was a drama all in my mind.

What a relief to let it go. I feel lighter. And happier. And like my clothes aren't out to get me!

She's so right, and, reader: I bought two of those sleeveless dresses, chicken flesh be damned.

DO YOUR BOOBS HANG LOW? CHANGING BREAST SIZE

AS WE GET OLDER, the tissue and structure of our breasts begin to change, once again due to our fluctuating hormone levels. As a result of reduced estrogen, the skin and connective breast tissue are less hydrated and thus less elastic. With less springiness, our breasts start to sag, and it's not uncommon for an older woman to have a significant change in her cup size. Sometimes it goes down, but more often it goes up. One friend has saved all her prettiest (and expensive) bras in the back of her lingerie drawer "just in case." For the last five years she's been wearing cheap stretchy sports bras because she can't quite face that her larger breasts are probably permanent. The increase is due to something called involution, where the milk-producing glands shut down and breast tissue is replaced by fat. Water retention and weight gain are also factors. Fat is softer than breast tissue, so our boobs don't feel as firm. I went through a period where my floppy breasts made me feel a little inhibited during sex—no sex on top in broad daylight, please!—but I've recently gotten over it. I mean, I figure I'm really lucky I still have my breasts at my age; I might as well be proud of them, slackness notwithstanding.

ODE OF WITHERED CLEAVAGE

When I saw it for the first time,
I was baffled that anyone would walk out her door
showing that—the vines, the snakes,
the ripples, the nest of nestlings' necks!
And to think that on an ancestor
of that—if withered cleavage is
a descendant of fresh, young breasts—
I had spent some early hours of my life,
learning to adore the creamy
moon. My mother's desire to be touched,
late in her life, was so intense I could
almost hear it, like a keening from the hundred little
purselets of each nipple, each like a
rose-red eraser come alive and starvacious.
And now my own declivity is
arroyoing, and if I live long enough

my chest over my breastbone may look like
an internal organ, a heart trailing its
arteries and veins. I want to praise
what goes one way, what never recovers.
I want to live to an age when I look
hardly human, I want to love them
equally, birth and its daughter and
mother, death.

—SHARON OLDS

LET'S GET PHYSICAL: EXERCISE MATTERS

WHEN I WAS FORTY-FIVE I proudly reported to my gynecolo-gist, Dr. Laura Corio, that I had become a SoulCycle addict, and she responded that she wasn't at all impressed. Apparently, at our age all exercise needs to be weight bearing, that is, with pressure on the feet! Being up on a bike was making me sweat and helping my heart, but not fighting bone loss or adding muscle. Around the same time, I developed that painful case of tennis elbow I mentioned earlier, and the result of both the conversation and the condition was that I decided to consult a personal trainer, Alejandra Belmar of Brooklyn's Everyday Athlete. Alejandra and her team whipped me into shape with strength training, and six months later I had lost seven pounds, my back fat, and my injury! One of the many things her team pointed out to me was that I'd spent years taking the latest trendy exercise classes where no one was really watching my form. I'd gotten lazy, and the result was inconsistent results and injuries. This was a wake-up call to take a new look at both my body and my routine.

According to a 2015 article in *Prevention* magazine, these are the six major workout mistakes menopausal women make, and I think I've made them all:

■ **You're a cardio addict.** Building muscle mass and increasing strength is imperative as we age.

■ **You stick with swimming and cycling.** Think, "Bones, bones, bones!" My trainer explained it to me like this: "Your bones get stronger when they feel they need to." If you don't lean on them, they won't improve.

■ **You're lazy.** You can rest when you are dead. This is not the time to take it too easy on yourself.

■ **You eat like a thirty-year-old.** Our aging metabolism has slowed down, so we need to eat less to maintain a healthy weight.

■ **You skip warming up.** Older bodies need longer warm-ups— we're creaky!

■ **You're your own coach.** Try learning some new tricks from a professional. If you can't afford a few sessions with a personal trainer, look for a small fitness class.

Like diet, exercise is not one size fits all, and you've been in enough dentists' waiting rooms and airplanes to have read all the conventional advice in magazines at least a million times by now, so I will try not to bore you here. The gist? You need to move your ass regularly, and stretch to stay limber, and keep your blood pumping, and maybe more than anything else, do it upright a lot of the time, because weight-bearing exercise is key at our age. Some of the most effective weight-bearing exercises include jogging, hiking, dancing, stair climbing, jumping rope, and tennis. (Speak with your doctor before embarking on a new fitness routine that includes weight-bearing exercise; you don't want to injure yourself out of the gate. This is crucial if you have osteoporosis. The National Osteoporosis Foundation says lower-impact alternatives such as using an elliptical machine or fast walking outdoors or on a treadmill might be safer.)

Also, if you've been sedentary for a few years or never exercised at all, you must get off to a slow start and, really—I can't stress enough how important it is—warm up before and cool down after. The American Heart Association calls warming up "a critical bridge" to harder exercise and says it helps prevent injury, especially as we age. The experts also report that stretching (once your body is already warmed up and your blood is flowing) can help prevent muscle soreness and help maintain overall range of motion. Consider investing twenty bucks in something called a foam roller, and then go on YouTube and learn how to use it. Those things are gold for aging muscles, ligaments, and fascia!

A strong case for exercise is made by the lovely people at the North American Menopause Society (NAMS), the country's most important organization of gynecologists, researchers, and other experts on the topic. In a 2017 paper with the unfortunate title "Weight Loss Actually Possible After Menopause" (they might as well have put the "actually" in all caps and thrown in a couple of exclamation points), executive director Dr. JoAnn Pinkerton emphasizes that exercise can be a solid alternative to hormone treatments. "Documented results have shown fewer hot flashes and increased mood, and that overall, women are feeling better while their health risks decrease," she says.

More research from NAMS concludes that as we age, we may get a bigger bang for our exercise buck. A study out of the University of Massachusetts Amherst presented in 2015 showed that some types of physical activity have a greater impact on body composition in postmenopausal compared to premenopausal women. "Across the board, for each measure of body composition, we found that light physical activity had a greater impact in postmenopausal compared with premenopausal women," says Dr. Lisa Troy, lead author. "We additionally found that sedentary behavior was more strongly associated with increased waist circumference in postmenopausal women. This is an important public health message because, as women go through menopause, physiological changes may decrease a woman's motivation to exercise. What we've found in our study suggests that doing even a little bit of exercise may make a big difference in body composition."

Did that mention of increased waist circumference stop you in your tracks? It did for me. First, there's the vanity issue: My friend Lisa recently called me in a panic to borrow something to wear before a wedding because although her weight hadn't changed, she couldn't zip up any of her fancier dresses that she hadn't tried on in a year or so. More importantly, an increasing waistline is linked to cardiovascular disease. The *International Journal of Obesity* found that waist circumference is a better predictor of heart disease in middle-aged women than body mass index. Estrogen loss causes cells to store more fat and slows metabolism. In addition to heart disease, the Mayo Clinic warns that a measurement of more than thirty-five inches signals a greater risk of other obesity-related illnesses such as diabetes and high blood pressure.

Jordan Metzl, MD, a highly regarded sports medicine physician, says research shows that women our age get the most benefit from exercise if they work out sixty minutes a day at least four days a week. (I can hear your groaning, and I feel your pain, and for what it's worth, I certainly *do not* do this.) He recommends plyometrics (jumping!) to develop power, coordination, and balance, in addition to a mix of cardio and strength training. On "rest days" throw in some mind-body and mobility work like yoga, Pilates, or tai chi. Something to strive for at least. Jesus, how hard do we have to work out to keep in shape? Has anyone noticed the paradox of aging and having a slightly weaker body but now having to exercise twice as hard to keep it going?! Sometimes I just want to take a nap!

Alas, all the experts seem to say the same thing, which is that an ideal regimen is one that combines cardio with strength training. The following list is compiled from a combination of the Seven-Minute Workout (which came out of an article from the American College of Sports Medicine *Health & Fitness Journal* but was then made wildly popular by the *New York Times*, and which I love and use when I'm traveling in particular) and tips from my own trainer, Alejandra, as well as just plain common sense. I can tell you that if you aren't doing any of these exercises at least a couple of times a week, you probably should be:

The Very Basics:
- Squats
- Lunges
- Bent-over rows
- Plank
- Side plank
- Push-ups
- Triceps dip
- Jumping jacks
- Abdominal crunch
- Wall sit
- High knees running in place
- Step up onto chair

Alejandra adds, "Whatever your exercise routine is, don't forget to add some HIIT. High-intensity interval training, which includes short bursts of intense exercise, followed by stretches of more moderate activities, has been shown to reverse the aging process. It increases our mitochondrial capacity—which helps the body create energy—by far more than other types of exercise, and also improves our insulin sensitivity, which potentially lowers diabetes risk, and increases ribosome activity, which helps build proteins that create muscle cells. All good stuff!"

A 2017 study published in the journal *Cell Metabolism* and conducted by the Mayo Clinic confirms that HIIT is by far the best anti-aging workout at a cellular level.

Let's acknowledge here, though, that there are times in our lives when we can't physically (injuries, illness, exhaustion) or just plain don't want to do endless squats or goddamn lunges, but we still know we need to do something. A possible answer? The ancient art of qigong! Just as this book was going to press my agent, Heather, became obsessed with China's three-thousand-year-old system of healing arts, also known as "energy arts." Qigong practice typically involves moving meditation, coordinating slow-flowing movement, deep rhythmic breathing, and a calm, meditative state of mind. Heather says, "Every part of my body had been hurting—my feet, my back, my jaw, you name it. My eighty-year-old father recommended a daily qigong practice. I started using some links I found on YouTube, and I swear, it's changing my life." Whatever works, right?

For me, what helps with both the boredom factor and the results is variety. I have to change it up constantly, or I find my body plateaus. I've been through every exercise trend there is, as I'm sure many of you have: yoga, tennis, barre, Pilates, Zumba, SoulCycle, personal trainers, running. After a year or two of any consistent routine or fad, I start to realize my ass is sagging more and I need to switch to something else. As of this moment, I'm running twice a week (by which I really mean shuffling, for at best two miles, with some walking interludes), seeing a trainer once a week (twice when I'm feeling either especially fat or especially flush) for weight training and form, and hopefully doing yoga once a week.

THE BENEFIT OF FITNESS TRACKERS (HUMAN OR MECHANICAL)

If you're having trouble getting motivated, I suggest one of two things: find a workout buddy—someone who will go to the gym with you, chat on the treadmill, hold down your feet for sit-ups, that sort of thing—or get the next best thing, a fitness tracker (they used to be called pedometers). You can find one on your iPhone or iWatch in the Health app, or you can buy any number of fancy gizmos to wear such as a Fitbit, Jawbone, or Nike FuelBand (one friend swears this is the prettiest and sort of looks like a high-tech bracelet, or at least that's what she tells herself) that will track your steps (aim for 10,000), calories expended, and even your sleep, depending on what features you want. I tried one for a while and it really helped me stick to a routine, and then I moved on to the next trend, whatever that was.

OUCH, MY KNEES! (BACK, SHOULDERS, ELBOWS, HIPS...)

SOME DAYS MY KNEES ARE FINE and then there are days when I truly feel physically like an old woman, like I can barely pick up a quarter if I drop one on the floor. If I say again that this is attributed to hormonal fluctuations, will you kill me? Sorry, it's true. Estrogen fights inflammation. In the *Menopause in an Hour* video series, Dr. Tara Allmen notes that aches and pains are very common. She also points out that after menopause, there's an increase in frequency and severity of osteoarthritis or degenerative arthritis (which is a common cause of joint disease).

To ease these aches and pains, experts suggest the usual: maintain a normal weight, exercise regularly, take 1,000–2,000 IU of vitamin D_3 daily. (D_3 is more readily metabolized into a bioactive form of D that is easily converted to its hormone form in the kidneys. It takes much longer to convert vitamin D_2.) According to the Arthritis Foundation, women with higher vitamin D levels are about one-third less likely to develop rheumatoid arthritis. Discuss supplements such as glucosamine with your doctor. NSAIDs (nonsteroidal anti-inflammatory drugs) such as ibuprofen can help, as can acetaminophen, but again, discuss how often it's safe to take over-the-counter pain medications with your doctor, because overdoing it can harm your liver. Also, drink a ton of water. I'm convinced that when I'm more lubricated, my joints hurt less.

The biggest thing within our control here is what we eat. I'm a sucker for the Whole30 program, or any of the anti-inflammatory regimens, because I notice that I feel significantly better when the majority of what I eat is simple proteins and vegetables. It's not the most sustainable diet, though, and in fact co-founder Melissa Hartwig doesn't even recommend that you do it endlessly. A less strict option might be the Mediterranean diet, one that is high in fruits, vegetables, legumes, and healthy fats (olive oil and nuts) and low in saturated fats and simple carbohydrates. Eating this way is reported to have anti-inflammatory effects as well as being loaded with antioxidants, which help limit the damage done to your cells by free radicals. A large, rigorous study published in *The New England Journal of Medicine* found that adopting the Mediterranean diet prevented 30 percent of heart attacks, strokes, and deaths from heart disease in people who were considered high risk (e.g., smokers, those with diabetes, those who were overweight). Plus you get a little bit of wine.

WHAT THE HELL IS THE WHOLE30 ANYWAY, NINA?

The Whole30 is my go-to diet plan when I'm feeling I need a reset. These are the basic rules: eat meat, seafood, eggs, tons of vegetables, some fruit, and plenty of good fats from fruits, oils, nuts, and seeds. Eat foods with very few ingredients, all pronounceable ingredients, or better yet, no ingredients listed at all because that means they are totally natural and unprocessed. No beans, no grains, no dairy, no sugar, no alcohol, no gluten. It's essentially the caveman diet in high heels.

Lastly, anything physical that keeps you in touch with your body and feels good is wonderful, whether it's massage, regular stretching, acupuncture, or physical therapy. Many women I know (who can afford it) turn to massage—myofascial work, deep-tissue massage, Swedish massage, craniosacral, whatever rocks your boat—to deal with menopause symptoms such as sore joints and muscles, as well as anxiety and fatigue. Putting yourself in someone else's hands, being taken care of, can also feel like a great relief. Any activity that increases your range of motion, eases postural restrictions, and helps you stay in touch with your body is a positive.

A flotation tank joint, an enterprise called Lift, recently opened in my Brooklyn neighborhood. For an introductory price of $75, I entered a small chamber full of highly salinated water, and I floated there, naked, for an hour. At first I thought it might be unbearable (I love baths, but I start to let the water out about two minutes after I've gotten in the tub), yet whether due to the isolation of the tank, or the salt, or the perfect temperature, I found myself luxuriating in the Zen of the experience, and before I knew it the subtle alarm was going off, telling me my hour was up. As I got dressed to head back out into the cold New York City winter, I reflected on the power of that hour: self-care, meditation, being alone with my body and my mind. It was good.

MY BODY, MYSELF: LOVING YOURSELF AS YOU ARE

All health begins with how we perceive
ourselves and our bodies.
—CHRISTIANE NORTHRUP

WRITING AND RESEARCHING this chapter made me dig deep into my own feelings about my body, and basically, I'm grateful it still works and I think I take it for granted far more than I feel self-critical. Sure I wish I looked like a twenty-five year-old, but that would be absurd, since I'm forty-seven. And I'm happy I can still run and jump and see myself getting stronger with effort, and God knows I'll be super-bummed when the day comes that I am weak and bed-ridden and unable to take a brisk three-mile walk.

I canvassed some girlfriends with the question, "What's bothering you most about your body these days?" and my friend Isabel's response was typical "At fifty-four, I actually feel like my body has held up pretty well. I wish my boobs had retained some of their fullness, but there's nothing else I really can complain about. It's the bigger things, what I think of as the fault lines—my chin, my wrinkles—that I can only address via surgery, and since I'm not willing to go under the knife, I just have to sigh and accept what is..."

A recent study published in the *Journal of Women and Aging* investigated body-image satisfaction in middle-aged women over fifty. Using a sample of almost eighteen hundred American women, researchers found that just over 12 percent (!) of the participants reported they were satisfied with their body the way it was. Aspects of their physical appearance that these women reported feeling unhappy about included their skin (80 percent), their stomachs (56 percent), and their faces (54 percent). Researchers also found that participants who had undergone cosmetic surgery were no more or less satisfied with their body image than women who did not have surgery. And, no surprise, in the group of women who did report satisfaction with their bodies, researchers found that these participants were less likely to have eating disorders and dieting behaviors.

About the findings of this study, lead researcher Dr. Cristin Runfola noted, "Of course the fact that so few women are satisfied with their body size is concerning. But we were interested in how some women remain happy with their size and shape given ubiquitous social pressures to retain a youthful thin appearance, and the influence of a multibillion dollar anti-aging cosmetic industry." Interestingly, satisfied women exercised more than dissatisfied women, and weight and shape still played a primary role in their self-evaluation. Weight-monitoring and appearance-altering behaviors did not differ between groups. What does all this tell me? Mostly what we already know: that women are enormously hard on themselves when it comes to appearance and that we have a lot of work to do in the self-love and acceptance department. I think by sharing how we feel with one another, we can edge closer to Dr. Northrup's goal of feeling like age-less goddesses.

BETTINA: *I'm more okay with my body image than I've been in a very long time. I work hard at it and still have anxieties about what would happen if I were to stop. But I have a history of teenage bulimia and though I sometimes think of it, I am pretty sure I'm past the point of acting on it. Which feels like a grown-up thing.*

I read a 2017 *New York* magazine article by journalist Marisa Meltzer, in which she discusses the new trend of not body positivity but *body neutrality*, and it both appealed and made sense to me, particularly as we age.

It's simple and obvious but bears repeating. Sometimes you'll lose weight without trying, and sometimes you'll gain weight without trying. Some days your lower back will feel like it was run over by an SUV and some days your breasts will feel perfect and remind you what it was like to be thirty again. The important things are not to delay your happiness until that magic moment and not to be so damn hard on yourself all the time. "Body neutrality isn't a license to throw in the towel, dive head-first into a pile of chips and give up on feeling healthy," writes Metzer, "but to move on from the mindset of needing to lose weight or worrying about what you see in the mirror to focusing on how you feel." It's about how you want to allocate your time and focus. Meltzer interviewed Ann Kearney-Cooke, PhD, director of the Cincinnati Psychotherapy Institute, who says, "Neutrality is the freedom to go about your day without such a strong focus on your body. We have only so much energy, where do we want to use it? There are lots of other things that need attention. You don't want to neglect your body, so you listen to it, and are aware of the function it serves." To which I can only say, *amen.*

I'm not saying you should give up on your dreams of having the body you want. I'm just asking, if you never get that waist, will your life have been a waste?

—CAISSIE ST. ONGE, *MEDIUM*, 2016

CHAPTER FOUR

(PARENTING)

A (NOT QUITE) EMPTY NEST

When your children are teenagers,
it's important to have a dog so that someone
in the house is happy to see you.
—NORA EPHRON

THIS HAS DEFINITELY BEEN my strategy. I got our dear beloved Muffin, a lab/pointer mix, when my eldest child was twelve. That was also the summer of my separation from my first husband, and the beginning of my experience as a single mother. My kids were twelve, eight, eight, and six.

It's ten years later now, and, Lord, how many parenting mistakes have I made since then?

Not all of us have had kids. Some skipped it altogether by choice or circumstance. Some are stepmothers and aunts. Some of us stopped at one, and others, like me, went all the way and had four or five. I don't personally know anyone who has actually birthed more than six babies, but of course you're out there. And for those of us who do have them, we started at varying times.

At forty-seven and with a fully empty nest, I'm on the young side.

I have (exhausted) friends who are in their fifties with kids in elementary school! There's definitely no one size fits all to this conversation, perhaps in this chapter more than in any other chapter in this book, but, since the majority of moms over forty are familiar with the joy and tyranny that are teenagers and young adults, that's where I'm going to start.

HAS IT BEEN EIGHTEEN YEARS ALREADY?

IF YOU'VE REACHED THIS AGE and don't know that clichés exist because they're true, let me enlighten you. One of the biggest of all is how fast kids grow, how parenting flies by, how the years just disappear. How dead-on all those statements are. It truly seems like yesterday that my babies were born and coming home from the hospital, that I was bathing their little bodies in the kitchen sink, that I was wrestling with strollers and car seats and finding babysitters and helping with science projects. And now—poof!—they're gone. Yes, they all managed to learn to read and write and do long division. And then suddenly they are driving, have pubic hair and breasts, and drink and smoke weed and have sex. They are my size or bigger, and there are whole huge parts of their lives that I know nothing about.

It's a monumental feeling—having the kids gone and staring down the rest of my life. I'm still in the throes of trying to make sense of it. My identity as a parent, and as a woman, has shifted seismically, and I'm still not quite sure what that means, or who I am, with them on their way. Sometimes I come home to my empty apartment and breathe a sigh of relief, and other times I walk in to all the quiet and a panic seizes me—"What now? What will I do with myself without them here?!"

But first, let's go back for a second: lots of my friends found the baby stage hard. Diapers, tantrums, the tedium of being at home with small children, the feeling that you'd never get your life back. I even have one girlfriend who swears that she almost died of boredom being a parent—*until* they became teenagers, when she started to enjoy it. Wow. Talk about the power of different perspectives! I was the opposite. A born logistics maven, and one who enjoys checking tasks off a list, I found having little ones almost nothing but joy. Or maybe it looks so easy in retrospect because I've found teenagers to be so incredibly hard? They were so darn cute when they were small. I loved their chubby little legs, their intoxicating smell, buying tiny clothes at Target. Sure the car seats sucked (at one point I had a triple stroller and three car seats; my back hurts just remembering it). But doing things like extracting snot from their stuffed up little noses— remember that weird rubber bulb?—made me feel capable and in charge. Meals, groceries, doctor appointments, babysitters, toys, bedtime reading. Check, check, and check. No problem.

Middle school is when things began to get rough. Suddenly everything got so complicated—the jockeying for social status and increasing demands for independence; their insecurities, first crushes, and budding sexuality; the Internet! By the time they were in sixth or seventh grade it was abundantly clear that the personalities and characteristics that were identifiable from day one had now coalesced into cogent beings who were marching about the world and getting bigger and stronger every day. My ability to control their lives was simultaneously dwindling and I started to stumble.

During that time, I was also splitting up with their father, so all my moorings were coming loose. My eldest turned twelve when we got divorced. Would my experience of those years have been easier if their dad had been around on a daily basis? Hindsight is always twenty-twenty, but I'd venture to say, "Hell, yes!" Not only was I a complete wreck, but we were all navigating a new dynamic, and the kids were figuring out how to manage (and manipulate) within the new system just as we were creating it. Messy for everyone.

Mothering adolescents while in the state of perimenopause is a whole trip unto itself. The ingeniously funny writer and performer Sandra Tsing Loh has a whole shtick on the "diminishing of the estrogen cloud," with the attendant exhaustion and moodiness, and how that directly correlates to us reaching a point where we really can't mother a goddamn second longer. I have had many a day recently when I'm standing in the kitchen and spy a piece of errant food on the floor—a hardened strand of spaghetti, a piece of broccoli—some scrap a mostly innocent (lazy, sure, but not trying to send me to the loony bin) kid has haphazardly let fall while cooking or eating, and I can feel the rage start to boil from my feet to the top of my head. It's as if the insult of mothering, the inordinately unfair burden of it all, has suddenly reached its zenith. Inexplicable rage, out of nowhere, is not uncommon in perimenopausal women, but if you're reading this book, you probably know this already.

Not to mention dealing with their sexuality. On a recent holiday break, every time I went into one daughter's room, I found an empty condom wrapper strewn on the floor. I happen to know that this young woman is on the Pill, so I wondered—why the condom wrapper? I asked. "Oh," she said. "X is a real rule follower. His mom told him to always use a condom, so he does." There could be far worse exchanges, but the thing is, no one truly wants to have this kind of bedside chat with her child. How I miss the days of cuddling up reading *Little House on the Prairie* together. I don't want to be imagining her in her room screwing her boyfriend every night, and I certainly don't want to be cleaning up her sexual detritus. By the way, she feels exactly the same. I remarried when this daughter was fifteen, and more than once she has alluded to the fact that she is completely grossed out by the thought of me having sex with this old man (her perspective, not mine) who now lives in our house. While I suppose I should be grateful that she's open with me, the subject makes us all squirm. It was all much simpler when I was the mommy and she was the child, and adult sexuality was not in the picture.

BIG KIDS, BIG PROBLEMS

THE HIGH SCHOOL YEARS WERE when I really felt I lost control, and I'm still in this phase.

As of this writing, my children are sixteen, eighteen, eighteen, and twenty-three.

Way too often they treat me like I'm essentially an ATM machine and the emergency contact to be called when there is a problem—and, boy, have I lived through almost every teenage problem you can imagine. Out of respect for their privacy, I'll put it this way: between my own kids and their friends, I've been party to shoplifting, arrests for open containers of alcohol in the park, teenage pregnancy, nude (and rude!) Internet behavior, school suspension, eating disorders, depression, anxiety, bullying, being bullied…and I'm still counting my blessings, thinking of all the ways it could be worse, and praying I make it through to that magical stage when science promises their frontal lobes will be completely developed without the ceiling completely falling in. It's terrifying.

When there is a crisis with teenagers, you wonder—legitimately—how much worse it might get. Is my daughter or son just smoking some recreational weed (I still call it "pot," to their chagrin), or will weed be the gateway drug to heroin? Is she mildly depressed the way I was at fifteen, or is she going to attempt suicide one day? Is his eating disorder something we can conquer, or will he be sick like this for the rest of his life? My girlfriend Kiki's son was on strict probation for five years from age nineteen to twenty-four for something really stupid but highly illegal, and she and his father lived in mortal fear of him screwing up and going to prison. The stakes are high, and so much of what they think and feel and do is hidden from parental sight. My rule of thumb is that, for all the stuff I know (and often wish I didn't), it's probably only about 15 percent of what goes on in their lives. In other words, I'm like an idiot savant, sensing my way from the periphery, armed with cash and experts and hard-earned wisdom, bailing them out royally at times, but often ignored and clueless. For a control freak like me, this is a very tough place to be.

THE HAPPINESS PARADOX

DOES HAVING CHILDREN make you happier? Not in the United States, it seems. According to a 2016 study done by the Council on Contemporary Families, comparing data from twenty-two European and English-speaking countries, American parents report being less happy than nonparents by quite a wide margin. In fact, we have the largest happiness gap of any of the countries studied. The best explanation for this difference is that our society's support for mothers and fathers is almost nonexistent, but the fact is that the difference shows up, albeit in smaller numbers, in much of Western society. Variations of this study have been done in numerous forms by myriad researchers, and the results are usually the same: childless people report being happier, and parents (deluded?) consistently say they can't believe it.

In her excellent book, *All Joy and No Fun*, journalist Jennifer Senior posits that day-to-day happiness is higher for childless people, but the happiness that parents feel is more of an abstract, long-haul happiness. Not only are American parents regularly stressed out by the lack of a comprehensive support system, they are riddled with anxiety about their own parenting choices. In a recent interview with the *New York Times*, Christine Gross-Loh, the author of *Parenting Without Borders*, who lives in both the United States and

Japan, said, "In Japan, my 6-year-old and my 9-year-old can go out and take the 4-year-old neighbor, and that's just normal." An American mother who gave her children that kind of freedom might end up being hauled into the offices of Child Protective Services. When *do* you let them walk to school alone? At what age are co-ed sleepovers allowed? Is it crazy to let eighteen-year-old Susie drive the family car to Vermont? With her siblings? So many nonstop decisions all the time. It's very hard to know what the rules are, and we're constantly feeling judged—by ourselves and by others—or making the wrong move. I think Senior's distinction between joy and fun is an apt one; when I imagine a life where I never had children, it feels as though my soul would be missing. It's almost incomprehensible to imagine my life without the deep satisfaction that loving my children has given me. On the other hand, is it *fun* being a mother? Often not at all, frankly.

The number of women who don't have children is higher than I would have guessed. According to data from the Pew Research Center, in 2014, 15 percent of women age forty to forty-four have never given birth. Of course, there's a big difference between being child-free by choice (Woolfer Carla told me she never once felt "the impulse" to have kids, and added, "None of my friends who are childless by choice regrets it") and being child-free by circumstance, either because of a biological or physical obstacle or because, like my friend Deirdre says, "I never met the right guy and by the time I did it was too late." I've been envious of child-free women who seem to have boundless energy for their jobs, social lives, and travel and say, "I love being an aunt—and then shutting the door." I've also stayed up all night drinking wine with and handing tissues to a late-fortysomething friend grieving that she would never have kids.

Note to mothers: talking about kids to a friend who has none can be a sensitive subject, so please use your brain. The same friend Deirdre said to me, "Nothing pisses me off more than people asking, 'Have you thought about adoption?' Of course I've thought about it! I decided I didn't want to go that route after much thought, so please don't bring it up like I'm clueless."

In 2013, an irritating *Time* cover story on "The Childfree Life" by Lauren Sandler caused a momentary stir. Illustrated with an attractive, affluent white couple lounging on the beach, the packaging and headline seemed calculated to pit mothers against "selfish" women without children (which wasn't the journalist's intention). Just like the age-old "mommy wars" (the tension between working and non-working mothers, which, sure, does exist, but not nearly as much as the media would have you believe), this was another cultural attempt to amplify differences between women, when in fact I'd argue that if you look beyond the superficial, there's generally more solidarity and common experience between us, both joyous and painful. Some women are single; some are childless. Others are divorced, and yet others are battling disease. There are a million ways to live our lives, and we're all wanting or lacking or suffering in some way. As much as anything, what has helped the women I know to survive, whether we are struggling to breastfeed baby twins, accepting a failed IVF treatment, breaking up, or mourning the loss of a beloved family member—whatever the obstacle—is the support of female friends. Childbearing status is irrelevant.

COPING WITH AGING WHILE BENDING OVER TO PICK UP THE LEGO BRICKS

ON A SLEETING JANUARY EVENING while writing this book, I organized a group of ten Woolfers for what we called a "Hormone Dinner"—an opportunity to sit down in an informal setting and ask ob-gyn Laura Corio absolutely anything we wanted about perimenopause and menopause. Over tequila and cheese, we got comfy by sharing stories and secrets (hot lube! who knew?). As the conversation turned to the subject at hand, someone pointed out that perimenopausal women have a ton in common (estrogen roller coaster, anyone?) with their teenage daughters, and how that makes for a complicated home life. Nods of commiseration all around, except for the two women in the crowd, both over fifty, who piped up that they each had toddlers at home.

In both cases they were unexpected pregnancies that had occurred the good old-fashioned way, through unprotected, impassioned sex. Even Dr. Corio, who has practiced for almost forty years, looked surprised (and impressed). Since I myself stopped having babies sixteen years ago, and feel vaguely nauseous at the prospect of getting pregnant now, I interviewed them to get a feel for what having a child was like in your late forties.

ALISON'S STORY

Alison discovered she was pregnant a couple of weeks shy of her forty-seventh birthday, around the time she was taking her eldest son on college tours. Five years before, her second child had died in a tragic rafting accident when he was eight. "Before my son died," she told me, "my husband and I did talk about wanting a third." Both felt they "weren't done parenting yet." Alison had fibroids, which were getting worse, and after three surgeries, she went to a specialist who said having a baby would involve a rigorous fertility treatment plan. "We didn't have the energy for many reasons and said forget it…and then, boom! I got pregnant." Although she had all the physical signs of early pregnancy, she barely believed it herself. "I did an at-home test and read the results wrong. I went to eat lunch and suddenly ran back to look at the stick and thought, 'Oh my God…'"

Although she had a long labor, she described it as the easiest of all her three births. When her baby was a newborn, she says, "I was much more relaxed; I didn't sweat the small stuff. I could see the whole trajectory of him growing up, so I felt like, "If he doesn't sleep through the night or throws up on me today, it's okay." Now that he's three, Alison doesn't feel the pressure to enroll him in a million activities. "He loves the park; I take him on his scooter." She says when she remembers all the classes she schlepped her boys to when she was in her thirties, she thinks, "Well, that was stupid."

Alison also describes her husband as being a more hands-on caregiver now that he's established in his career and not feeling the need to work late and on the weekends. "He's more committed," she says. "Part of that is also losing a child." She told me the hardest part of being a parent of a young child at this age is losing some of her and her husband's freedom to be spontaneous and seeing their friends taking off to travel. (She also said with a smile, "And my friends are so jealous about my sweet and cuddly boy!") When I asked her about the "terrible twos," she answered her little guy never had them. "He's so much fun; he's brought life into our house."

MEG'S STORY

Meg and her husband married in their midforties and hoped to have children. "We tried on our own," she told me. "We knew there was no guarantee." After six months, they saw a specialist, who found that Meg had only one fallopian tube and an abnormally shaped uterus (as she describes it, "the worst kind"). He recommended IVF. "I had a poor tolerance for medication, a funky uterus, and only a fifty percent chance of carrying to term." She also weighed in the odds and risks of having a baby at forty-eight, deciding the chances of getting pregnant were infinitesimal. "IVF centers don't even keep data on women over forty-five. My husband and I felt like we had a good life and we would roll with it."

Meg was experiencing perimenopausal symptoms when she discovered she was pregnant. "We spent a few weeks looking at each other saying, 'Holy shit...really?'" They had just bought a fixer-upper house, full of lead paint. "I didn't want to get overexcited; I was violently ill and it was a struggle to get through the day. I lost eleven pounds in the first six weeks." Even when she made it through the first trimester, she was still cautious because of all the risks. "Until they handed me a healthy baby, I couldn't get on the roller coaster." At about thirty-two weeks, she thought, "Okay, this is going to happen." Meanwhile, she was couch surfing while her husband worked like a

WHAT WOULD VIRGINIA WOOLF DO?

madman on the house and living on protein shakes, canned peaches, and frozen waffles—the only foods she could keep down.

Week forty rolled around and she didn't go into labor, so after a few days, she was induced. After twenty-eight hours of laboring, she had a C-section, during which the anesthetic "crapped out." (Yes, you read that right.) But there came "this amazing baby girl." She was determined to breastfeed and said she was "that crazy lady who makes the nurses bring the baby every two hours after having surgery." When they were allowed to go home, it was bliss; the baby was "serene and snuggly." But twelve days in, Meg got a kidney infection, spiking a fever, and was rushed to the emergency room. "My husband was bursting into tears and finally breaking down because he's got this newborn and thinks I'm dying!" She spent three days in the hospital, with her husband riding back and forth on his bike to fetch pumped breast milk so he and his sister could finger feed the infant with a tiny tube.

Finally back at home, Meg was relieved that her daughter still latched on. However, she felt traumatized and exhausted but couldn't sleep. "Finally, I started sleeping again. It was kind of comical. I'd wake up hearing a strange noise and realize, 'Oh! It's the baby!'"

Despite the incredible stress of her pregnancy and birth, now that she's a mom, Meg says she feels more confident and competent than she would have if she had had a kid in her twenties or thirties. "I realize I'm not perfect, and that's being human." She acknowledges that perimenopause adds its own special challenges. "My husband and I aren't as intimate as we'd like. We're lying there on the couch falling asleep at nine thirty—and my vagina is as dry as the Sahara desert! Not to mention that my now four-year-old is wide awake and staring at us."

But then she describes the poignancy of what she refers to as her "amazing gift." She says people can be judgmental about whether it's ethical to have a baby at fifty. Meg and her husband realize that they will be in their seventies as their child finishes college and use that as a reminder to focus on what's important in life. "When everybody is grumpy and I just want the kid to go to bed, I think about that."

I have to admit, hearing these stories made me want to have a baby immediately! For about three seconds. The idea of how calm I'd be, how wise. I could do everything right this time, and they are so darn cute. But then I look up from my desk and see the dog. Muffin and I are here at home, alone, and it's so very quiet. When I finish my work I can do whatever I want...take a bath, meet my husband for dinner, curl up with a book. I think I've earned the rest (and frankly, I think I need it, whether I've earned it or not) and will hold on to it. But God bless these ladies.

BEFORE I FORGET...THE BRIGHT SIDE

WHEN THINGS ARE PEACEFUL, I still marvel at my kids' charm and smarts and adorableness, just like I always have. How wonderful it is to see my son, my baby, now over six feet tall and 180 pounds, hold the door open for me when we walk into a building. Or to hear him speak knowledgeably about literature. The heart soars! My eldest and I don't agree on a lot of things politically, but I'm still so damned impressed by the way she can spout figures and facts and argue her case. Her poise is remarkable.

One of the nicest things about my children is that they genuinely love one another and are super-close. They laugh together, they *get* one another, and they adore being together. I realize this isn't always the case with siblings, and I don't know why it happened here, but it's beyond touching and gives me great comfort. I love knowing that they will have one another in a deep and sustained way long after I'm gone. The flip side of this is that I often feel left out. I'm the adult they love but don't really want to hang with. I have many a vacation photo of my four big kids walking arm-in-arm as a phalanx down a foreign street, me straggling behind with the camera. When they are all at home, I'll often come into the kitchen at midnight to find the four of them, with various friends and lovers, all laughing, eating pasta, and playing Monopoly in teams. If I hint about joining in, I'm met with an awkward silence. They usually try to be polite, but they obviously prefer one another's company to mine. Sigh.

I'm guessing (praying?) this will change, and it will be one of the perks of getting older. My kids will come back to me. A therapist once told me that it's perfectly normal, even "right," for kids to want nothing to do with their parents from around fifteen to twenty, and then they return. I can already see it with my eldest. At twenty-three there's a real shift in maturity, and even a budding appreciation and respect for her lowly parents. And I swell with pride watching her actually being an adult.

IT'S OFFICIAL: FRENCH WOMEN ARE BETTER AT EVERYTHING

A FRENCH WOOLFER, GERALDINE, RECENTLY pointed out that there is no translation in French for the word "parenting." This came up during a conversation over coffee about the intense pressure American mothers put on themselves when it comes to raising kids. She asked, "When did this quest for being the perfect mother start?" The literal answer is that the word "parenting" didn't appear in the United States until 1958, according to the Merriam-Webster dictionary, and became common parlance only in the 1970s. She went on to say:

> Because my mother was not like that at all; she did not blame herself if we were doing something wrong. She kept saying, "You were lucky to be born in a privileged family. You have no excuses. If you mess up, that's your problem; it's your life, not mine." She was nice and kind, but we were in charge. And it made things easy. I don't know if French mothers do better than American mothers, but I know for sure that we don't feel as guilty, which makes our lives as women way easier (more time for your marriage, among other things). My two kids went to school when they were two and I loved it!

Vive la France, as they say, but have the French never heard of Freud? Of course everything is my fault! That said, I do try to embrace the nonhelicopter model. I'm not an overinvolved parent in many ways—I didn't do their homework for them ever, I let them travel alone and take the subways young, I generally believed that conveying trust in their own innate capability to figure stuff out was key—but that has its own drawbacks and dangers.

No matter how hard you try, as the poet Philip Larkin says:

They fuck you up, your mum and dad.
They may not mean to, but they do.
They fill you with faults they had
And add some extra, just for you.

But they were fucked up in their turn
By fools in old-style hats and coats,
Who half the time were soppy-stern
And half at one another's throats.

Man hands on misery to man.
It deepens like a coastal shelf.
Get out as early as you can,
And don't have any kids yourself.

—PHILIP LARKIN, *THIS BE THE VERSE*

GRAB YOUR BAGGAGE, WE'RE GOING ON A GUILT TRIP

WHY DO WE FEEL GUILTY? To me, it's obvious. From the time the children are shooting down the mini-slide at the playground until they are walking onstage to accept their diplomas, all eyes are on Mom. Dissecting mothers for their flawed parenting and the impact it will have on their offspring is something of a national pastime (see "It's Official: French Women Are Better at Everything" earlier in this chapter). It begins in utero (no sushi! no wine! don't stress! bad mom!); continues through birth, which ideally—so as not to traumatize the infant—would be 100 percent natural, attended by a midwife, in a bathtub, and accompanied by whale song; and goes on forever. Unless fathers do something really egregious (like incest), they get infinitely more leeway. Don't believe me? Consider the flip side. Have you ever noticed when a dad does something that would be considered normal for a mom, say, bake a birthday cake, take a sulky tween shopping for a bar mitzvah party outfit, or actually play at the playground, everybody oohs and aahs like he's some kind of humanitarian hero? This may be changing with younger Gen Xers and millennials being stay-at-home dads or at least trying to split the parenting fifty-fifty, but still, there's just no comparison with the burden mothers bear in the guilt game.

I feel all the time that if I had done a "perfect" job (whatever that means), my children would be perfectly happy and good and successful in every single way. Yes, I do realize that sounds ridiculous, and yes, I am familiar with D. W. Winnicott's 1953 theory of the "good-enough mother." (If you aren't: "The good-enough mother...starts off with an almost complete adaptation to her infant's needs, and as time proceeds she adapts less and less completely, gradually, according to the infant's growing ability to deal with her failure.") This is basically a psychological theory designed at least in part to defend the ordinary mother against what Winnicott saw as the growing threat of intrusion into the family from professional expertise. It's a term that has gained casual popularity, and you can see why—it ever so slightly lets us off the hook. Most of us can say, "I'm sure I was good enough!" But when you are in the trenches, and your kid is miserable or making major mistakes or doing actual harm out in the world, it's very hard not to feel like it's all your fault. "If I hadn't gotten divorced/if I'd gone to more of Sally's gymnastics meets/if I'd cooked dinner more often/if I'd read more books aloud at bedtime/if I drank less/if I wasn't always so worried about money/if I didn't hate their father so much." God knows there are a million "ifs" running through the heads of most mothers.

I nodded in silent agreement as my friend Magda vented to me over the phone recently. "Being a mother is impossible. I'm a doer and a problem solver, but neither seems to apply to raising my kids. They are who they are, no matter how much you love them and how much you do for them. They make small mistakes and huge ones—you can't anticipate this. I'm always thinking, analyzing, and worrying about the next thing. I don't ever feel settled or calm. My children are my life, my love, my everything, but they are also killing me slowly... Was it stupid to have them? Yes! Would I do it again? Yes!"

All we can really do in the face of self-blame and guilt is face our regrets, reconcile them with the reality of our flaws, and accept that we truly did the best we could.

A NOTE ON OUR OWN MISERABLE CHILDHOODS

If you have never been hated by your child,
you have never been a parent.
—BETTE DAVIS

ALL OF US REACT TO (and/or model, for better or worse) the ways in which we ourselves were parented. This is a depressing but unavoidable fact of life. In my case, my parents were both self-absorbed artist-intellectuals who were too caught up in their own pursuits and dramas to pay me and my younger brother much attention. So they ignored us and traumatized us with their extravagantly complicated lives (adultery, violence, rages) but were also inspiring and glamorous in their intelligence and humor and daring work. A mixed bag, just as most people would probably describe their childhoods. I was left on my own a lot as a kid and forced to be extremely independent early. A therapist would say (and has said) that my "emotional needs were not met." Now, as my kids near adulthood and as I continue to wrestle with the vexations of my own psyche—my relationships with them, with myself, with the world—I have to accept the ways in which I passed this legacy on. I wasn't always the most present parent. I was distracted and melodramatic and caught up with my own stuff. I was a bit larger than life, which was probably both inspiring and daunting. Do I have to go on? The ways we can beat ourselves up is endless...

It's worth thinking about all this and acknowledging our foibles. Hopefully it's never too late to apologize for the ways we may have screwed up. Woolfer Elena and I recently had an email exchange about our kids in which she offered this:

> My kids are my everything and the huge challenges they've presented have only helped me grow and learn about myself. For me, therapy is an invaluable source of guidance and clarity, greatly enhancing my adult relationships with them.

It was a helpful reminder to me that there's always work we can be doing on our most dear relationships.

MY OWN MOTHER'S EXPERIENCE OF THE EMPTY NEST

It is refreshing to me to feel every now and then that the caretaking is finished, and I am free again! Hard to digest, I'm sure. But true. Every step away is both sad and liberating. For you. For me. We will change our relationship a million times as the years move on. And that is because we are committed to change and not to static energy. It is our way. Not many people want growth the way we do. Most people want to settle, find a place of comfort and cling to it. But in all our years of living that is not how we structured things. We lived together, yes, but it was always understood that as some new interest emerged, some new adventure presented itself, it was to be taken advantage of, and if it brought change in its wake, so be it. In that sense I have always loved your separateness from me, always cherished that I was in fact simply your custodian, so to speak, for a period of time until you had your own wings. I still feel that way. That your flying through life on your own pleasure, your own wits, your own steam, is the true excitement, your true living. And my own flying an equally important thing. And that ultimately it is only delight in another that holds one, that is captivating, all else must be a respect for their freedom. Don't worry though, as all requests are honored if possible. You only have to say when you need me, momentarily, to offer pure mothering. It is, after all, and after all these years, quite deeply ingrained in me and has given me such an intense pleasure.

—KATHLEEN COLLINS, IN A 1987 LETTER TO ME
WHEN I WAS EIGHTEEN, MONTHS BEFORE SHE DIED

This is so beautiful and so complicated. My mother was a remarkable woman, and she was also quite selfish in some ways. To me, this is a great example of how mixed our legacies of parenting and love invariably are.

HAVE YOU SEEN MY BOUNDARIES?

But kids don't stay with you if you do it right.
It's the one job where, the better you are,
the more surely you won't be needed in the long run.
—BARBARA KINGSOLVER, *PIGS IN HEAVEN*

EVEN THOUGH WE'RE DOOMED TO MAKE mistakes and feel guilty (at least if we're American), establishing boundaries is crucial to one's sanity, and more than ever, as we and our children are getting older. When I see some mothers (and some fathers) still essentially wiping their teens and twentysomethings bottoms for them, it makes me sad for everyone. How on earth are these young people going to manage out in the real world? According to the Bureau of Labor Statistics, about 40 percent of those who start college won't have finished by the time they hit thirty. It's no wonder that some kids can't cope with college, or move back home the minute they graduate. And the poor moms are making themselves absolutely nuts with balancing busy jobs, worries about money and retirement, managing their hot flashes, and still endlessly catering to and fretting over their lazy-ass kids. The buck's got to stop somewhere, don't you think?

Partly it's complicated because the parents and the kids are doing a push-pull dance where no one is quite ready to let go. My kids complain that I treat them like babies, and I sigh and protest that they want to be treated like adults but still act like babies. Woolfer Susanna summed it up: "It's weirdly irritating when they only care about their teen world and you want to shake them out of the innocence to which they cling, staunchly."

One of my daughters, when she comes home on break from college, will often text me in the middle of the day and say, *"Can you drive me to X?"* When I ask when, she responds, *"Now."* It's mind-boggling. Does she, at eighteen, have no sense that I actually have a life and responsibilities and a packed schedule? Does she think, in some corner of her brain, that I'll just be sitting in my room for the rest of my life, waiting patiently to satisfy her every need? When I'm in a good mood this strikes me as funny, and even endearing, the way they think they should still be at the center of my world when in fact they live elsewhere and are legal adults, and *I'm* trying hard to now be at the center of my own world! But when I'm in a bad mood it can make me enraged. The entitlement! And then after my pique subsides, I drop what I'm doing, grab my car keys, and we're off.

When they are all back to their lives at school and work and I'm alone again, I find I'm mostly loving my newfound freedom. Then a week will come where I feel aimless and sad and I realize that it's about my empty nest, that I desperately miss my babies. Our children are our anchors in so many ways, and while having them grow up and go is necessary, it's also a very real loss. I'm no longer the center of their lives (well, psychologically we could dispute that, but I'm no longer in charge, anyway), and they are not the organizing principle of mine anymore. That's an enormous shift. I spent twenty-two years with children underfoot, and now, just like that, they're gone. The opportunity for reinvention is exciting, but sometimes I worry.

It's challenging enough to make huge shifts in your life when you are young and idealistic and lusting for life, but reinventing yourself when you are tired, achy, jaded, and unpredictably incontinent can be downright terrifying.

WEANING KIDS FROM THE FINANCIAL TIT

I GREW UP IN A household rich in culture and poor in cash. I heard the phrase "we can't afford it" frequently and was well aware of domestic stress when the washing machine broke or the pipes froze, because I knew my mother usually couldn't afford to fix those sorts of unexpected things right away, and it was scary for her. I had paying jobs from the age of thirteen. I babysat, cleaned, had a paper route, and that advanced into working in the local library, waitressing, and telemarketing. And then my mother died when I was nineteen. Hence I became accustomed, from a young age, to handling and managing money. I was paying all my own bills before I turned twenty and even supporting my younger brother financially.

My own kids have had a more privileged upbringing. Unexpected repairs have never been a financial strain, they've gone to great schools, and my ex-husband (who also grew up with considerably less) didn't think they should have to have jobs until they were adults, and I went along with that. We started modest allowances when they were in middle school, and each child was expected to carry out certain tasks (as much as I may gripe, my kids are all whizzes at cleaning the kitchen) in exchange for the doled-out weekly money.

I hear stories of kids in their twenties who come back home to live, and it scares me. According to the Pew Research Center, in 2014, for the first time in more than 130 years, adults ages eighteen to thirty-four were slightly more likely to be living in their parents' homes than they were to be living with a spouse or partner in their own house-holds. To which I can only say, "There but for the grace of God go I." I know people who are paying their adult kids' rent and credit card and cell phone bills and making their doctor appointments, and honestly it sends shudders down my spine. How will they ever learn to take care of themselves? My friend Katie is apoplectic when she comes home after work to find her that her twenty-seven-year-old son and a bunch of his friends have been smoking pot and drinking beer in the trashed living room all afternoon. Still, she lets him live there in his childhood bedroom, rent-free, and provides a full fridge and the Internet. Granted, I probably grew up too fast, but since my kids hit late adolescence I've been pretty fixated on making them financially independent.

My bottom-line rule is that in college and during the summer, my kids have to work for their own spending money. After tuition and room and board (which, let's face it, is already like renting Versailles; they are so lucky I'm footing the bill), it's reasonable to expect them to contribute. I love to take them shopping for clothes occasionally when we're all feeling warm and fuzzy, but I firmly discourage the casual "Mom, can I have some money...?" question that was de rigueur in high school. After my eldest graduated from college last year, I thought long and hard about the appropriate way to help her in this major transition to adulthood. I also realized I was setting a precedent and whatever I did would be expected by her younger siblings. Their father and I decided we would send her a modest amount each month to supplement her income for one year, and after that, she was on her own. We also told her we wouldn't be paying for graduate school. That was a hard one, but I don't want any of my kids just going to more school because it's the easy choice. If she does go to graduate school, perhaps later we would help her pay off loans, but the financial burden would be primarily hers.

You know what? She rose to the occasion and made me feel like a good mother to boot. At twenty-three she shares an apartment, has a job, makes her own doctor and dentist appointments—even checks the oil in her used car at regular intervals. Admittedly, there have been some emergency calls and ones from which maybe some other parents wouldn't bail her out (like when her beloved pet rabbit, Gretel, needed a very expensive hospitalization—*ugh*), but they have been rare. I'm proud of her and I think she feels proud to be taking care of herself.

We all have different values and expectations, but most parents want their children to grow up and be independent. I don't want to tell you what to do and not do with your kids. So much of what we feel when we talk about money is not really about money, right? It's about our childhoods, what we need to feel safe, our sense of worth in the world. I value independence. I want to know that my kids can take care of themselves in case I'm no longer around. So that's me.

Here are some tips provided by the Colorado Society of Certified Public Accountants:

- Talk to your kids about money. Don't think about it as a taboo subject.

- Don't be afraid to say no. Some children have been conditioned to think that their parents will keep providing forever because there have never been boundaries on spending. Kids have "wants" that then become "needs." Parents give their kids more toys or clothes than they need. That turns into expensive hobbies, cars, credit cards. After years of no financial limits, children will not know the difference between a need and a want and will have no sense of financial responsibility or independence.

- Decide what your limits are and make a plan. Put it in writing. Have a family meeting and discuss your expectations and let them know you want them to grow up to be financially independent adults.

- Before they go to college, kids should have their own bank account and understand how to read the statements and what fees and overdraft penalties there may be. Ditto if they have a credit card.

- Teach them how to create a budget and come up with long-term goals for saving money—even a small amount.

- Explicitly state that your financial support is limited, and do not reward their dependency. Do you really want to be supporting your kids (even grandkids!) when you are trying to save for your own retirement?

■ There will always be unexpected events—car troubles, health issues, bad jobs. Decide in advance how you want to respond to your kid's crises and how much money you are willing to lend or give.

FIRST DEPARTURES

I CRIED PRETTY MUCH NONSTOP the summer between my oldest child's high school graduation and the late August day when the whole family (ex-husband included) drove in a two-car top-heavy caravan to take her off to college. I was forty-two at the time and devastated. My own mother had died soon after I left for college back in 1986, and I'm sure that played a role in my grief. Because I never had a mother after the age of nineteen, I couldn't imagine that my daughter could have one. What would that almost-adult relationship look like? But I think my sadness was also just the universal first loss of a child going out into the world. Had I done a good enough job? Would she be okay? How would I bear missing her so very much?

I came home after that drop-off and walked by her empty bedroom for the first time. The room had been cleaned, and also emptied, since she took all her choice possessions with her to Boston. It looked like a hotel room, and the sight brought up fresh tears. But I did also notice that her bathroom, which I pass every day in the hallway leading to my own room, was spotless too, with gleaming tiles and the notable absence of dirty towels and mounds of cosmetics... and therein, a gleam of light in all the darkness.

By November, I was a happy camper. What you don't realize when it's first happening to you is that *they never actually go away*! They're not gone; they're just in another place. It's just a new normal. They text, they call, they need advice, they ask for money. You send gifts, and sheets, and before long, they visit. As the weeks wore on, I had to admit to myself that she was ready to go. That whole last summer at home was full of restless, bored energy. She had lived her childhood here and was now itching for new adventures and to be on her own, to find her own way. It's the natural order of things, and as one friend said, "Would you rather have them living in your basement in twenty years?"

THE TEN BEST THINGS ABOUT THE EMPTY NEST

1. Not worrying all the time about where they are. Even when they are home on break (this is also true for my eldest, who has graduated from college!), I can't sleep until I know they are safe and sound in bed. But as soon as they are out of sight, away at school, that worry magically disappears. I have no idea what time they come home, and I don't fret about it. I've heard I'm not alone in this; it's a time-space continuum mothering mystery.

2. When I come home at the end of the day, everything is exactly as I left it. No piles of shoes and coats and backpacks in the hallway, no papers on the dining room table, no mess in the kitchen. Or, all those things, but they are mine, and they don't bother

me because I left them there. No blaring music, no crowds of teenagers, no incense burning to cover up other smells. Just an empty, clean apartment and a friendly wagging dog. This is such a treat, I can't tell you.

3. The fridge is semi-empty in the perfect way. No tubs of cream cheese, no bagels, no enormous bottles of orange juice. I can fill it with fruits and vegetables and choice proteins, or fancy vegan desserts, or just bottles of club soda.

4. The companion to numbers two and three is that grocery shopping goes from being a thankless Herculean task ($400 trips to Costco followed by the job of unloading and unpacking, only to have the food gobbled up in a few days by children I don't even know, who barely grunt at me as I pass through the kitchen) to being a sort of Mary Tyler Moore adventure! I breeze through the local shops, picking up just the small things that my husband and I need for the next day or so. I feel Parisian!

5. We can walk around the apartment naked! We can have sex in the living room! Never mind that we don't actually do this. The *feeling* of that kind of freedom goes a long way.

6. I don't have to worry about people rummaging through my nightstand, desk, closet, or medicine cabinet, borrowing my clothes, using my lipstick, judging my sex toys, or stealing my once-a-year pack of cigarettes.

7. *So* much less texting! I still text with my kids most days, and I love that connection, but I'm no longer texting constantly:

    "When will u b home?"

    "Where r u?"

"Will u walk Muff?"

"Has Muff been fed?"

"Have u done your HW?"

"college essay!?"

"Have u found a summer job yet?"

"No, u cannot stay out another hour"

"NO, I really mean it"

Or the classic combo, which I must have typed ten thousand times over the teenage lives of four kids:

"How/where r u?"

8. No lost socks and bras. When the kids are home my husband and I are *constantly* "losing" these items…

9. We don't run out of milk for coffee.

10. No contact highs.

THE TEN WORST THINGS ABOUT THE EMPTY NEST

1. No one around to walk Muffin.
2. Missing hugs.
3. Missing watching them sleep.
4. No family dinners.
5. Not seeing and talking with their interesting friends.
6. Not learning about the latest music and shows.
7. No technology help!

8. No one to give me fashion feedback.
9. Not knowing when they get new piercings.
10. Knowing I'm now officially old.

THEY'RE BACK...

ANOTHER FIRST IS THE FIRST TIME they come back after they've been away, and if you haven't been through this yet, let me prepare you: it's not a piece of cake. Anyone who tells you it is, is either Mary Poppins or on a lot of Xanax.

Here's how it goes for me: I'm super-excited. Christmas/Thanksgiving/a special birthday weekend is coming up, and a kid or many are coming home. I prepare by doing a huge grocery shop and buy and cook their favorite foods. I make sure their rooms are spotless, with fresh sheets and towels and maybe a scented candle. I fantasize that we'll watch movies together and get our nails done.

Then the day arrives. I trek to the airport or the train station, usually in horrible traffic or rain (because it's always winter when this first happens, and we live in the Northeast), and there are usually delays. I've sat for up to three hours in my car at LaGuardia Airport more than once since my son left for school in Minnesota. But I'm happy to do it, because I so love my boy! Said kid arrives and looks happy to see me. Big, warm hug, kisses all around. My sigh of relief to have him or her back.

Usually within minutes, maybe ten or maybe twenty, I say

something innocent that yields a grimace. It could be a well-meaning question about the latest love interest, or about schoolwork, or about summer plans. Somehow, I've offended. Then the child in question usually plugs his or her phone into my Bluetooth (often disabling mine, which will take me weeks to figure out how to reinstate) and starts blasting music, which sometimes I love, but sometimes it's Drake or Nicki Minaj and the lyrics are so vulgar that I can hardly think straight after two minutes. Then he or she starts texting furiously, surely making plans for that night and days ahead (or maybe just chatting with his or her siblings to complain about Mom), which will barely include me.

I think you get the point. I probably don't need to detail the piles of dirty laundry that come out of the suitcases, or the clothes that never once go into empty drawers or closets and become monumental towers of mess on bedroom floors. Streams of friends, also home on break, come over and eat all the food. It's typical for me to grocery shop every day when the kids are home. Yes, they are charming and I like to hear how they are, but they also drink all our wine and beer (are they even legal yet? probably not, although they all have fake IDs) and flick ashes in the garden, and even though the dishwasher is running constantly, no one ever empties it and the sink is almost always full of dishes. And the bathrooms? I won't even go there.

Then they leave again and I am bereft.

CHAPTER FIVE

(BEAUTY)

MIRROR, MIRROR...?

What's the matter with looking seventy-five?
—MARY BEARD

IF YOU'VE EVER SAT BY the bed of an ancient dying person, it's staggering to ponder the growth and disintegration of the body from birth to death. As we age, we literally shrink and shrivel up, and frankly, the process is often not so pretty. Aging is indisputably cruel in certain ways, and the changes to our appearance, while superficial, are dramatic. More than halfway along this trajectory, I'm plenty aware of the changes in my own looks and the waning of my physical beauty. My breasts sag, and one of them has a permanent divot from a surgical breast biopsy I had in my thirties (benign, knock on wood). Oddly, luckily, I'm not yet gray, but of course that will come, and my hair has become duller and thinner than it was for sure. My face, with new lines and changing contours, seems to be aging at a precipitous rate. And no matter how hard I exercise, my body has lost its tautness; soon the best word to describe my skin will be "slack." This is all an unavoidable reality: each of us will eventually, if we live long enough, come to resemble our mothers, and then our grandmothers, and then we will die.

Given that this is a natural progression, and one that we actually hope to experience as long as we can, I feel pressure to be a good role model to my daughters in this regard. I don't complain to them about being old, or about my lines and scars or general feelings about my fading looks. I try to model strength and grace and pride in my appearance because that is what I hope for them at every stage throughout their lives. That said, I'd be lying if I said I'm not *noticing* what's happening to me, or having twinges of sadness about it. When I think about why I'm feeling this way, it really is about mortality and the realization that we're all going in one direction. Recently I went to a neighborhood cocktail party full of people I've known casually for almost twenty years. I noticed age spots on more than one hand, and receding gums, and straw-like gray hair. It was disconcerting to me; I admit it. Fading looks point to fading life, and that can be a bitter pill to swallow.

Women are not alone in facing the melancholy trio of beauty, aging, and death—men feel it too—but for us, because of societal expectations and pressures, the changes in physical appearance that happen at midlife often come with feelings of panic, even for those of us who never seemed all that invested in our looks to begin with. This conundrum comes up all the time in the group. One day my friend Jan, a woman who has sworn her whole life by an ascetic facial regimen of Ivory soap and water, looked at herself in the harsh early-morning light of winter, and all of a sudden saw in the bathroom mirror droopy and asymmetrical eyelid folds and ever-so-slightly bumpy undereye pooches. Her heart gripped in fear, she called me in a near-hysterical state, suddenly fixated on finding a "miracle" eye cream, no matter the cost. I totally relate to her crisis: the lines under my eyes are more like creases or indentations—I'm not sure how else to describe them. They look like I slept on a pillow full of rocks in the back of a truck for ten hours. They started only under my right eye about two years ago, but now are under both, and these aren't bags; they are funky patterned lines and I have no good goddamn idea what to do about them. Probably nothing will make a whit of difference, but I'll surely continue to slather a range of high- and low-end products on my face in the eternal hope that something will slow down the ravages of time. Do I feel panicky? No. Distraught? Only if I think about it too much.

Let's face it: we can be ambivalent, we can alternate between acceptance, resignation, and fight, but the bottom line is that how we look matters to most of us in one way or another. If beauty weren't a huge issue, we wouldn't be spending nearly $150 billion a year on anti-aging products and treatments in the United States alone, according to industry analysis by Zion Market Research, or getting our faces coated in acid, injected with botulin and derma-fillers, and even getting sliced, stretched, and stitched back together again.

Of course, physical beauty is defined by different cultures and different eras in different ways. In the United States right now there's a premium on the beauty of extreme youth—especially for women. The whole idea that men just get better-looking as they age, while women get ugly, is definitely embedded in our cultural subconscious. When did you last hear of a woman over forty being described as "more distinguished"? A few years ago, *New York* magazine published a telling infographic on the relative ages of cinema's leading men and their female love interests. In *Dark Shadows* we saw Johnny Depp (forty-eight) paired with Bella Heathcote (twenty-four); *Flight*'s Denzel Washington (fifty-seven) was paired with Kelly Reilly (thirty-five). At the 2016 Berlin International Film Festival, Meryl Streep, one of the great exceptions to the aging-out-of-being-a-leading-lady rule, said that when she was in her thirties, she didn't think that she'd have much of a career after forty and the roles she saw mature actresses being offered were mainly hags and witches. Writer and actress Annabelle Gurwitch, in her book *I See You Made an Effort*, describes the erasure this way: "I'm fifty-two, which is actually eighty-two in actress years," adding, "Being a woman over fifty in Hollywood, I could commit any crime with impunity, because I'm completely invisible."

Flip through the pages of any American fashion or beauty magazine and you may feel a twinge of alienation or insecurity. Once I hit a certain age, the editorial models looked like they were playing dress-up in some very wealthy middle-aged woman's closet. What teen buys a $2,000 blazer or purse? The beauty and skin-care ads are even more jarring. In the UK, Helen Mirren (who is in her early seventies) is a spokesperson for L'Oréal's anti-aging products, which she agreed to do only on the condition that her image would not be retouched (bravo her!). In the United States, the same products are represented by Julianne Moore (who is in her midfifties), whose freckles and lines have been airbrushed into an unblemished white oblivion. There's also what I think of as the "three-crow's-feet rule:" Check out any picture of a celebrity spokesmodel of a "certain age" (which could be as low as thirtysomething). She's allowed three little smile lines around the eyes, and the rest of her face and neck is digitally sandblasted. Granted, even a heavily retouched Moore is far more relatable than the baby-faced models barely out of adolescence who are generally used to promote skin care and cosmetics. There's such a disconnect between the ideal audience—grown women with buying power—and the way the models look in the pages or in TV ads.

So, we're dealing with the inescapable reality of our changing looks, and balancing that against cultural pressure to either try to stay young-looking or age "gracefully" and accept turning into wallpaper. There are definitely bigger problems in the world (climate change! opioid addiction!), but still, our beauty and sense of attractiveness are things we think about, grapple with, and have to make personal choices around. On the one hand, we're lucky that women today have so many choices about how to approach this thorny spot. But ultimately, however we may want to mollify ourselves or not, the hard, cold reality was nicely summarized by Annette Bening, who said, "I don't really have a choice. I'm getting older."

ARE MY BOTOX TREATMENTS CONTRIBUTING TO THE "NEW NORMAL"?

ONE DAY WHEN I WAS a mere thirty-eight, one of my then elementary school–aged daughters said to me, "Why do you have so many lines between your eyes? They make you look so angry all the time." Sigh. Maybe because I'd just gotten divorced and was more worried than usual about my looks, this comment sent me running to my beloved dermatologist, a woman named Dr. Rose Ingleton who also happens to be a friend. Rose concurred that I had "particularly strong facial muscles." She pointed out that every time my face went into any kind of consternation, I looked a bit like a pug. (She didn't use that exact word, but in my keyed-up state, that's how I took it.) She offered to shoot me up with Botox and I readily submitted to the needle. (Yes, it hurts slightly, but not more than any other shot, and you use ice for a few minutes afterward; it's minor in terms of discomfort.) And once I started, well...a little between the furrowed brows turned into tackling the deep lines across my broad forehead, and then eventually the smile lines by my eyes, and so on. A slippery slope, indeed.

Botox is made from a purified version of the toxin secreted by the bacteria that causes botulism, a rare but potentially fatal paralytic illness. We aging women have this stuff injected by medical professionals into our countenance to cosmetically remove wrinkles by temporarily paralyzing our facial muscles. The procedure is insanely popular—according to *Time* magazine, Botox use is up 759 percent (I had to triple-check that stat; it doesn't even seem like a real number, it's so big) since 2000, and we pay a lot of money to do this depending on what part of the country we live in, how resistant our muscles are, and how many areas we want to tackle—anywhere from $200 to $1,400 every three to four months. Personally I love the stuff, but am I embarrassed that I use it? Absolutely. Do I wish I would stop? Yes. Am I planning to stop? Not quite yet. My rationale? I have really intense furrows between my eyes and a huge forehead with deep horizontal creases. (Or at least I think I do—it's been a while since I've seen them in full force!) My wrinkles make me look old and grumpy. After Botox, my face is placid and flat, more youthful, and that makes me feel good out in the world. That said, it's an addiction I'm conflicted about and embarrassed by. It's a sick use of money (there are starving kids all over the world and a million other actually important uses for thousands of dollars a year; yes, I do know this), and it also does feel to me like an insult to feminism. Who am I trying to look like? Why can't I just be me? Also, I can't do this forever. I'd look an idiot with a perfectly smooth face at some point, so my modus operandi at the moment is to try to go longer between appointments and to ride out seeing my lines emerge. It's a process...

One has to be super-careful about overdoing any of these interventions. A few years ago I went out for lunch with a particularly savvy and truthful girlfriend. As I sat down in the restaurant, the first thing she said to me was, "You're overdoing it on the Botox. Your face looks like the tundra." Ouch. With any intervention, we run the risk of going too far and looking ridiculous. Let us never forget the cautionary tale of Jocelyn Wildenstein, the billionaire who is reported to have spent more than $3 million on plastic surgery. Her face is so deformed that she barely looks human, and in fact the New York tabloids nicknamed her the "Catwoman." This is something to avoid, ladies, and we need to help one another out here.

One of my best friends, Lucy, is firmly in the anti-cosmetic-surgery camp and has always vehemently said that she would never "stick a needle full of poison in her face." Even though there have been remarkably few reports of serious adverse effects reported to the FDA over the fifteen years Botox has been approved for cosmetic use, the idea (poison injected into your face for the sake of beauty) freaks her out and she very reasonably feels it might create an unhealthy illusion of what an aging woman's face should look like. However, after Lucy moved to Los Angeles from the East Coast at age fifty, she admitted the pressure was intense, even for her. And I've since seen signs of wavering resolve. The last time we spoke she said, "I'm hiding my wrinkles under my bangs but I'm starting to cave." Personally I'm selfishly praying she hangs on, because I'm counting on her being inspiration for me to stop one day.

IF I COULD TURN BACK TIME: THE MAGIC OF RETIN-A

There is no such thing as a "miracle cream," but Retin-A is about as close as you can get. It seems to be one product that we mere mortals and dermatologists can all agree on. My friend Sarah's dermatologist, Kristen Miller, MD, who promotes a no-frills skin-care routine, says, "It's the only thing that works." When Woolfers are sharing skin-care recommendations, Retin-A pops up a lot, along with sunscreen, sleep, and water. In one of the many threads about skin care in the group, Andrea said, "Genetics is number one; sunscreen is two. I add in Retin-A to help correct the fact that I was very bad about number two. Honestly, if I had a time capsule, I would go back and wear sunscreen all the time." Sabine agreed: "As a journalist who has done stories on it and researched it: Retin-A. Nothing else. And scrubs of course."

Not to be confused with retinol, an ingredient used in many anti-aging products and cosmetics, Retin-A used to be available only by prescription (until 2017; see next paragraph). Both are retinoids derived from vitamin A and both promote skin cell turnover, but the latter is far more effective at tackling fine lines, rough bits, and age spots. Retin-A can also be used to treat acne because it keeps your pores from clogging with dead skin.

Retin-A is pricey, about $150 a tube, but you need only a tiny glob per application and it lasts for months. In 2017, the FDA approved the first over-the-counter Retin-A cream, Differin, for acne. A number of Woolfers reported that their dermatologists recommended it off-label as a much cheaper but effective alternative.

Warning: Retin-A can also be irritating. Especially when you first start to use it, you might experience burning, redness, peeling, and itching, pretty much the opposite of what you were hoping for. If you can stick it out for a couple of months, you should be rewarded with smoother, clearer skin. You can mix a bit with moisturizer and use every couple of nights to minimize the side effects as your skin adjusts. Some dermatologists also suggest breaking in your skin with gentler retinol first. Retinoids can make your skin more sun sensitive, so always apply a day cream with SPF.

To frame the debate in a slightly different perspective, I was comforted after a conversation with highly regarded New York City dermatologist Dr. Doris Day (that is her real name, I promise), who sees it quite differently: "The reality is that Botox and the other FDA-approved neuromodulators are drugs with an outstanding safety profile. Any drug is a poison when used incorrectly. This is one where we know down to the molecule how it works—we know how long it takes to take effect, how long it takes to wear off, and we place it where we want it to work. It's actually not meant to freeze anything. When done well, it helps to retrain muscles so that the negative muscles pulling down become weaker and allow the opposing lifting muscles to take over. You *can* move all your muscles, but the way you *do* move can be more beautiful and you can actually age better. I consider this to be true natural and graceful aging and I don't think it's anything to be embarrassed about for anyone." So stick that in your hat!

FRAXEL, JUVÉDERM, PEELS ... PICK YOUR POISON

I'M NEITHER A PHYSICIAN NOR a bona fide beauty junkie—I have friends who are much more up on the latest offerings from the fanciest doctors and aestheticians. But I'm also no slouch in this department. So here I'll give you a broad survey, as well as my thoughts, on some of the cosmetic adventures we can avail ourselves of in the quest to keep up (that is, if we are so fortunate, or desperate, to spend so much hard-earned cash in this way).

There are a lot of in-office facial treatments you can get, all of which aim to brighten and exfoliate your face and empty your pocket of anywhere from $200 to $1,200 a pop. There are so many treatments, and more coming out every day, but here's a rough summary of the landscape, in order from least invasive to most:

- **Dermaplaning.** This method of exfoliation consists of using a ten-gauge scalpel (inward scream!) to gently scrape off the top layer of dulling dead skin cells in order to reveal a smoother, brighter complexion. I've had this, and I liked it. It's win-win because the blade also removes unwanted facial hair!

■ **Microdermabrasion.** Treatments use a minimally abrasive instrument to gently sand your skin, removing the thicker, uneven outer layer. This type of skin rejuvenation is used to treat light scarring, discoloration, and sun damage and can smooth the appearance of stretch marks. I've also had this—my dermatologist offers a kind called a SilkPeel Microderm with Dermalinfusion, which involves a wand that feels like a wet vac, and it sucks all the crap out of my pores, then infuses my skin with whatever it's lacking at the time of the treatment (salicylic acid for acne and clogging, a skin brightener, antioxidants, or hydration). My face definitely looks brighter for a week or two afterward.

■ **Peels.** There are in-home peels, and then there are in-office peels, which range from mild to quite extreme. Aestheticians can apply vitamin C peels or mild acid peels as a part of your facial; then there are more serious chemical peels, which involve physicians applying alpha hydroxy acids (AHA), salicylic acid (a beta hydroxy acid, or BHA), trichloroacetic acid (TCA), or phenol to the skin to get a deeper peel. A chemical peel enhances and smooths the texture of the skin and is an effective treatment for blemishes, wrinkles, and uneven skin pigmentation. But the effects are short-lived—a few months at best—so you have to keep it up, which just means more expensive maintenance.

■ **Fillers.** As we age, our faces lose subcutaneous fat. This means that the facial muscles are working closer to the skin surface, resulting in more apparent smile lines and crow's-feet. The skin also is stretching (losing its elasticity), of course, which contributes to everything seeming to go south and an overall loss of facial volume. One answer, also not cheap, is injections of dermal hyaluronic acid fillers; some of the names you may have heard include Captique and Elevess (neither of which are popular in the United States), Belotero, Restylane, Radiesse, Hylaform (an old-fashioned collagen product, no longer available in the United States), Juvéderm, and Voluma. Basically it's like silly putty is injected into your face (to plump thin lips, enhance shallow contours, and soften facial creases and wrinkles), and then the doctor mushes it a little into the right position. If you're lucky, it lasts for many months and gives you a little satisfaction.

Note: this is where I get off the bus. I've done all of the above, and none of the below. But again, no judgment.

■ **Thermage.** Radio-frequency waves can target droopy skin, but I hear it burns like hell. Treatments such as Thermage work by delivering sound waves deep into the skin, causing microscopic fissures that stimulate collagen production, which in turn firms up loose and sagging areas (face, jowls, neck, knees, and so on). The results are impressive—most patients see significantly tauter skin within six months—but the procedure can be hard to endure. There's also the nonablative eTwo laser, which directs a much milder combination of radio-frequency and infrared-light pulses into the skin. The results are reputedly comparable to Thermage but not as painful.

■ **Laser treatments.** Even more expensive and painful but still a step or two away from plastic surgery are Fraxel laser treatments. It's a procedure that pokes microscopic holes in your skin so blemishes like sun spots, leathery bits that don't clear up the way they used to, wrinkles, acne scars, enlarged pores, and so on essentially crisp up, shed off, and heal over. I'm curious but was scared when I read reviews of treatments that mention "ice packs," "numbing cream," and "emptying your calendar so you don't have any social events for at least two weeks" as well as a sensation that one friend described as having your face bathed in hot sauce. How people have the fortitude to endure three appointments to complete the annual process/torture, I don't know. There is, though, a more mellow version of Fraxel called the Clear + Brilliant laser, which uses the same technology as Fraxel but is milder. There is virtually no downtime. The trade-off is that you have to do about three sessions of Clear + Brilliant to approximate the results of one Fraxel session. It's supposedly good for those who want the results without the downtime.

■ **Varicose vein removal.** I will admit to being lucky here. I may have a higher genetic risk of breast cancer because my mother died of the disease, but we do not have varicose veins in my family. Many of my beloved girlfriends have undergone all sorts of hideous treatments so that they can feel sexy on the beach, or just plain old climb out of bed nude. You start with your dermatologist, but depending on how far you need (or want) to go, you may wind up in the care of a vascular surgeon. Sclerotherapy is usually the first stop. It involves an injection of a solution (generally a salt solution) directly into the vein. The solution irritates the lining of the blood vessel, causing it to collapse and stick together and the blood to clot. If that doesn't work, there's sclerotherapy using some sort of detergent solution that is foamed and then injected into the veins, and then there are laser surgeries, catheter-assisted procedures using radio-frequency or laser energy, high ligation and vein stripping, ambulatory phlebectomy, and endoscopic vein surgery. *Ugh.*

THE DEEPEST CUT: PLASTIC SURGERY

MORE THAN 125,000 FACELIFTS are performed each year in the United States. According to the American Society of Plastic Surgeons, in 2015 they were the sixth-most performed cosmetic surgical procedure. (If you are curious, and of course you are, the first five, in reverse order, were tummy tucks, eyelid surgery, nose jobs, lipo, and—drum roll—at number one, breast augmentation.)

I haven't done anything [in terms of cosmetic surgery], but who knows…When you've had children, your body changes; there's history to it. I like the evolution of that history; I'm fortunate to be with somebody who likes the evolution of that history. I

think it's important to not eradicate it. I look at someone's face and I see the work before I see the person.
I personally don't think people look better when they
do it; they just look different...And if you're doing it
out of fear, that fear's still going to be seen through
your eyes.

—CATE BLANCHETT, *VANITY FAIR*, FEBRUARY 2009

Cate sounds a tad holier-than-thou here to me. Personally, I'm afraid of surgery and scars, so I won't be having any cosmetic surgery ever. But I will surely try other fillers/lasers/God knows what before I'm dead. Facelifts are among the most polarizing issues with regard to beauty and aging, and personally my motto here is, "Live and let live." Where I draw the line doesn't have to be where you draw it, and I think we should drop the judgment.

In the spring of 2017 the ever-hilarious *New York Times* columnist Joyce Wadler wrote an essay called "Swear You Will Tell No One" in which she announced to the world that she just had a facelift, and then proceeded to mock herself, and us, for all the subterfuge women go through on this front. She writes:

Heaven forbid someone figured out I just had surgery
to look better.

This makes no sense. People in this country yap
loudly on their cells about the kind of sex they've had.
They have affairs and put photos up on Facebook,
where their husbands or wives can find them. They

refuse to stand up and let people get past their seats at the movies. They work in customer support for Verizon.

I just wanted to get rid of my jowls and chicken neck.

That said, let's be real. Having a facelift is not exactly nipping into Sephora for a new lipstick. There will be pain, swelling, and a lot of bruising. You'll be in recovery for a good two weeks and, as one director of plastic surgery acknowledges, not yet ready for "primetime—such as a wedding or high school reunion—for one to four months." (According to the American Society of Plastic Surgeons, the procedure will also set you back about $7,000, and that's just the surgeon's fee; anesthesia and hospital room not included.) Consider why you want a facelift. If you want to look eight to ten years younger, that will probably happen. But if you are suffering from overall low self-esteem, a facelift may not help. A 2015 study published in *JAMA Facial Plastic Surgery* found that after six months, the impact of a facelift on a patient's self-esteem was negligible. In fact, for women who had high self-esteem before going under the knife, it was *worse*. Also there's the problem that apparently a few years later, you'll probably need to do it again. The skin starts to sag in strange places, and more surgical upkeep will be recommended. Rose explained to me, "The facelift just buys you about ten years before you start to see renewed aging. Then you might need a re-tuck." This sounds very Frankenstein to me, and something I'd like to avoid. But if you want to go this route, I'll happily go to a spa and sit by your side during recovery.

Another perspective, from a Woolfer:

> ***JONI:*** As a ghostwriter specializing in celebrity memoirs, I sit across the table from a lot of plastic surgery—good, bad, and ugly. The work seldom looks as pretty as the owner thinks it does, never looks as good in person as it does on camera, and usually ages into an ongoing maintenance lifestyle until you're looking at a Frankenstein construct of a woman who could have been stunning if she'd been allowed to age gracefully. I'm not judging women who get plastic surgery, but I'm sure as hell judging the culture that demands this of women and the doctors who profit from it.

LONG IN THE TOOTH

AROUND AGE THIRTY-EIGHT, I STARTED noticing that eating salad was a bit of a minefield. Have you experienced this too? It's called receding gums, and it's very common as we age. The gums diminish, and as a result, there is a bit of a gap that forms between the tooth and the gum, and that space is a great place for food to hang out. So you've eaten a salad, and you're gabbing away, and your teeth are covered in bits of kale and carrot. It's gross. Very unattractive. Very much a sign of aging.

I started asking around, and my friends gave me their tips:

- Overzealous brushing is a problem, so start using an electric toothbrush, which provides a more even pressure. Check!

- Try a Waterpik. Yes! My mother had one! Now I know why.

- Try pulling with coconut oil. An Ayurvedic approach, oil pulling is an oral detoxification procedure that is simply done by swishing a tablespoon of oil (typically our beloved coconut oil, but you can also use olive or sesame oil) in your mouth for ten to twenty minutes. Hmm...does that sound like a long time to be swishing oil in your mouth? Does to me...

- Carry floss in your purse at all times, and use it!

In any case, I ran off to my dentist, a man who is ten years older than me and whom I've been seeing since I was twenty. Marty gently said, "When we're not as young as we once were, these things start to happen, " and went on to explain the term "long in the tooth." Then he bonded my two front upper teeth for $800. Bonding is the application of a tooth-colored resin material (using adhesives and a high-intensity curing light) that fills in the gaps between your tooth and the gum. The materials are essentially glued to the tooth and sometimes come off and you have to do it again. It also needs to be done carefully, because you don't want the bonding itself to accentuate the problem; that is, push the gums farther away. Hopefully this will do the trick. What you really don't want to need is a gum transplant or skin graft, which sounds truly icky and painful and is one of my greatest dental fears for sure.

Woolfer Sharon had one, and here's her grisly tale:

> My oral surgeon told me that I had to have the graft-ing surgery, due largely to overzealous tooth brushing and flossing over the years…It wasn't fun, but if you don't do it when you need it, you can have bone loss and lose the tooth. I'm glad that he didn't scrape from my own palate because it hurt plenty in the one place, but if you don't harvest from your own mouth, you have to use a cadaver…which disgusted me no end. I've named that section of my gums "Uncle Frank" in honor of the anonymous donor.

Jesus. Scraping, cadaver, bone loss, harvest…I may faint. On top of all this, the recovery is hell. You can't brush your teeth for two weeks and have a hugely swollen face for days. Sounds excruciating.

On the more mundane side of dental issues, there's also plain old tooth discoloration. I have two upper baby teeth that never fell out, and weirdly they don't have adult teeth above them, so if they ever do get super-loose, I'm going to need implants! Oh no! But in the mean-time, as they hold on, they are noticeably more yellow than the rest of my teeth. I just live with it, but it's not so pretty. Once or twice in the last decade I've gone to one of those offices for a cosmetic whitening process (another few hundred dollars out the window for vanity), and each time I felt slightly perkier for about a week.

CREPEY NECK SKIN?

BELOVED DEPARTED NORA EPHRON FELT famously bad about her neck, and we get it; we all live in fear of having turkey neck. Is there anything to be done when it starts to happen? Again, my bestie derm Rose says that the options for treating skin laxity on the neck include stimulating tightening and collagen production with (1) radio-frequency heat (such as Thermage or the EndyMed device), (2) ultrasound heat (such as Ultherapy), or (3) a neck cream formulated to tighten and smooth. Botox injections are sometimes used to treat neck wrinkles too. And of course there's always the option of wearing a turtleneck and calling it a day.

NOT BY THE HAIR ON MY CHINNY CHIN CHIN

NORA FELT BAD ABOUT HER NECK; I feel bad about these fucking chin hairs. I keep tweezers everywhere: in every purse; in my medicine cabinet, of course; in my nightstand; and best of all, in my car, where the light somehow never fails to expose new growth I've missed (and this is particularly dangerous when I'm supposed to have two hands on the wheel of the vehicle). Despite the vigilance, it seems like nearly every day a new crop of the wiry little buggers sprouts. This is a very common complaint of middle-aged women everywhere, and in most cases our shifting hormones are to blame.

In the mirror at home, I have to put on my reading glasses when I pull out the tweezers to examine my face for rogue hair growth. It's not easy: I tilt my head up, nudge my glasses down my nose, and aim awkwardly to hit the exact combo of positioning that allows me to see what's going on along my jawline and under my chin. I always spot a few—so dark and so thick, like evil little blades—and slide them out like a pro. And then, the next day, or the day after that, I'll be sitting at a red light and glance at myself in the rearview mirror, and whoa! Suddenly there are like six new invaders, some as long as a centimeter, and I'm horrified to realize that I've been walking around like this—a woman with a beard.

It actually gets worse. As one of my girlfriends recently said, "It's bad enough *having* the chin hairs; the bigger problem is stopping yourself from touching them in public." Ah yes, I know that problem well. Like, when you're in a meeting or at a party and you casually brush your chin only to feel a hard piece of stubble there? And then you keep touching it, sort of fingering it, as if contemplating trying to yank it out right then and there? *In front of a room full of people.* Embarrassing and déclassé? Understatement. It's but one of the many beauty indignities that await, I'm sure, but so far it may be the one that gnaws at me the most.

BEYOND THE TWEEZER

THERE'S ELECTROLYSIS, waxing, and laser treatments, and I have friends who swear by using a razor. It apparently does not cause stronger hair growth and does not somehow result in you looking like a man with a five-o'clock shadow (contrary to what our moms told us about shaving our legs when we were twelve). I'm not sure why, but trust me. My girlfriends don't lie.

My go-to system for now, however imperfect, is a major investment in Tweezerman brand tweezers (definitely the best) and also in a little gizmo called Tinkle (easily found on Amazon, and yes, it really is called Tinkle) that is basically a lady razor that looks more like an eyebrow shaper. It's shaving that doesn't quite feel like shaving. Very ladylike, and at roughly six bucks for a multipack, one of the very few and very best beauty bargains you'll ever come across.

SORRY, CAN'T MAKE IT...THE HAMSTER'S SICK (AND OTHER LAME EXCUSES)

Nature gives you the face you have at twenty;
it is up to you to merit the face you have at fifty.
—COCO CHANEL

Have you ever skipped an important event because you felt ugly or old or fat? I find the idea of missing out on a graduation or wedding out of shame extraordinary. I sometimes have pre-party jitters, and I know women go on diets or pop their Botox cherries "to look good

---

in the pictures," but actually staying home? The more people I talk to about these changes we deal with as we age, the more I hear stories about pulling a dress out of the closet for a big do, finding it doesn't zip up anymore, and calling the host to tell her you are "sick." Or backing out of attending a twenty-fifth high school reunion because you feel overcome with embarrassment about your crow's-feet and wobbly upper arms.

My friend Lorien was freaking out about just such an event—a reunion. She'd ignored the previous ones, but number twenty-five was a milestone she wanted to mark. However, as the date approached, she became woozy with anxiety about seeing her old boyfriend, a guy who had abruptly dumped her for another girl toward the end of senior year. He had been a beautiful young man, a youth out of a Caravaggio canvas: dark curls, full mouth, deep-set hazel eyes. Lorien is an accomplished person; she heads a nonprofit, runs half marathons, and is the mother of two fabulously sassy daughters, but still, she was afraid to see the look on this guy's face when he saw her after all these years.

She started to dread every Facebook notification about the reunion weekend's planned activities (the usual stuff: family bowl-ing, eighties dance party, etc.). Like any good friend, her old bestie Elizabeth insisted that she show up and promised to be her wing-man, have Xanax on hand, and even bail if it was awful. Worst-case scenario, they could go get drunk at the skeevy dive bar that used to serve them when they were underage.

When Lorien arrived at the first night's reception, she nervously scanned the room for Pretty Boy. She didn't spot him at first, but then did see an oddly familiar bald guy with a fat neck and a tight, shiny suit...

Lesson? All of us are aging, and surely life is too short to let that fact keep you from celebrating the years you have left with the peo-ple you love.

EYELASH EXTENSIONS—YES, EYELASH EXTENSIONS

THIS IS MY FAVORITE beauty-enhancing trend of all time. Five or six years ago, I was playing tennis at nine a.m., and my doubles partner showed up looking like she was either off to Cinderella's ball or moonlighting as a Vegas showgirl. I asked, "Why on earth are you wearing so much makeup?" and she said, "I'm not wearing any; I just had my eyelashes done." I'd never heard of such a thing and pressed her for details. Untold thousands of dollars later (I refuse to add it up), I'm a bona fide addict. Every three weeks I go to a salon in SoHo, where they rub my feet for free while a woman glues on fake eyelashes, length twelve for me, C curve, as opposed to J. For me, who hardly ever wears makeup and whose natural lashes are stubby and straight, this has been the glamour pièce de résistance. Hubby number two thinks they are fabulous (and was slightly scandalized to learn they are fake), but I will admit that my ex-husband once told me I was seriously overdoing it and referred to my lashes as "that fur on your face." But he's my ex, after all.

There's also Latisse, which used to be prescription only, but you can now buy online, and lots of women who don't want to trek to a salon every three weeks (or fork over all that cash), but do want in on the super-long-lash trend, use it regularly. Apparently it's great, despite the small blindness risk (yes), but if you've never seen the hilarious You Tube video mocking it, I suggest you take a look (search "Lashisse from FOD Team"). Talk about fur!

FIFTY SHADES OF GRAY HAIR

Sometimes I think that not having to worry about
your hair anymore is the secret upside of death.
—NORA EPHRON

I DON'T GET THE CONVENTIONAL pressure about women need-ing to cut their hair after a certain age. It's another one of those things that strangers (and mothers) feel entitled to opine on. For some peo-ple, there's an idea that, like some items of clothing (short dresses or skinny jeans, for example), long hair isn't "age appropriate." It's not professional; it's too youthful; it's "witchy"-looking (ah yes, the ubiquitous trope of grown women being likened to nasty witches—if only we had magic powers). Some friends who have chopped off their hair have noted, after the fact and much to their chagrin, just how strongly it was related to their identity and sexuality. I'm forever try-ing to grow my own shoulder-length hair longer. To me, women over forty with long hair look sexy and strong, like lady Samsons.

Even more hotly debated is whether to go gray or hit the bottle. At forty-seven, I consider myself incredibly lucky to not yet dye my hair, and mostly I'm grateful because I spend so much time and money on other maintenance stuff (nails, waxing, eyelashes) that I feel like a regular trip to a colorist could very possibly send me over the edge. That said, I will inevitably go gray. Everyone's hair follicles contain a fixed amount of melanin cells (colored pigment), which eventually get used up. The age you go start to go gray is linked to genetics, race, and environmental factors, but about half of all people have a significant amount of gray hair by age fifty.

What will I do? I'm 98 percent sure I'll color it. Why? To look younger. I would never lie and claim an age younger than my true one, but I'm also not yet so psyched to proclaim with my hair, "This woman could have grandchildren." I admire the attitude of Woolfer Dana, who says, beaming, "My daughters refer to my gray hairs (of which there are many) as 'power sparkles.' But no, I'm just not ready to give up the dye. When will I stop? I don't know. I have many friends who have gone gray and look fabulous, so it's not that I disapprove." There's also the reality for many women (and men too) of feeling like we need to dye our hair just to "stay in the game," whether it's about competing with younger folks at work or getting back into the dating scene. Another friend says, " I imagine I'll stop when I get really sick of the effort, time, and cost. I'm guessing that for me it will be a gradual slide, like the Botox and everything else. I'll do it 'til I get too tired, too old, or too broke."

Going gray is a scary ordeal for some, to be avoided at any cost (and that cost could be well over thousands of dollars a year if you regularly go to a professional stylist). But for other women, it can be an exhilarating way to declare their maturity and wisdom and also look quite glamorous. Recall the late Susan Sontag's dramatic skunk stripe or Emmylou Harris's glowing silver mane. One way to tackle the transition is to start playing with color in general. Go magenta! Try a green stripe! Give yourself permission to experiment a little, and see what happens.

ELIZABETH: *I was recently inspired by my gorgeous, foxy, dear fifty-three-year-old friend, Vivian, to dye my hair blue-black. Don't know why I waited this long to play with hair color (I'm 50). It's been so much fun to have a new look and preen a bit. My husband, friends, and colleagues love my new hair—mostly because I love it. Pretty sure I'm now getting the eye from perky waitresses, who give me the "cool older woman" look I give older women. The looks make my husband jealous from time to time.*

Gray hair is also having a moment, with women in their twenties going silver (which I see as more of a fad than an homage!), but the majority of us women over forty are still hitting the bottle pretty heavily. According to a survey by Procter and Gamble, more than 65 percent of women have dyed their hair in the last year. Compare that to about 10 percent of women in the 1950s. My friend Grace jokes, "I can be flabby or gray, but not both." In her book *Going Gray: How to Embrace Your Authentic Self with Grace and Style,* Anne Kreamer argues that using hair color does the opposite of what we're hoping to achieve and is actually detrimental to our confidence (note a theme here; this is the same argument raised against plastic surgery). She decided to quit dying her hair after seeing herself in a photo standing between her blond daughter and her gray-haired friend. She writes, "Examining that snapshot made me think hard about who I was and who I wanted to be. Would I continue holding on to some dream of youthfulness or could I end the game of denial and move more honestly into middle age?"

My fear, as with all these beauty rituals (eyelashes, facials, nails, waxing), is that once you start dying your hair, it becomes a trap. If you decide to go natural, the gnarly part is the transition. I'm sure some women can work it, but several inches of gray with dyed ends is a hard look to pull off without the help of a hat for a year or two. You can talk to a really good colorist (though of course, it's not really in any stylist's financial interest to encourage a woman to stop dying her hair) or consult any of numerous Facebook pages or blogs such as those created by the Silver Sisters, a group of elegant dames including Cindy Joseph, whose modeling career took off only when she turned gray at forty-eight.

My friend Rebecca, fifty-five, is taking the gradual route. She, like most gals I know, has been dying her hair for close to twenty years. Her usual color is auburn, but recently, she's been going lighter and lighter and is now a strawberry blond that looks beautiful with her light brown eyes. She explained to me that (as a white woman), "As we get older the color contrast—dark hair, pale skin—starts to look sort of grim; it's better to let everything kind of mesh together." Well, whatever the logic, I've actually never seen her look more stunning. And it's a great transition to gray. She's going to get used to the paler color and then allow herself to slide right into au natural.

HAIR LOSS

IN THE BREASTFEEDING AFTERMATH of my first pregnancy, I remember combing my hair in the shower and watching fistfuls of hair come out of my head. Horrified and scared, I consulted my doctor and learned that this hair loss was a "normal" result of nose-diving estrogen levels after childbirth and was reassured that it would pass and all would be well. Fast-forward twentysomething years, and guess what? My estrogen levels are diving again, but they won't be bouncing back this time. And the hair loss is happening again! My shower wall looks like abstract art every morning. Woolfer Andrea, who used to have curly, thick brown hair like mine, says, "It feels like I have about forty hairs decoratively arranged on my head." There are a lot of reasons for hair loss, but the hormonal shift of menopause is a big one. Most women around fifty start to notice that their hair is losing both volume and shine, and I am definitely one of them.

If you are pulling enough raw material for a luxurious bird's nest out of your brush regularly or see that your part is getting wider or your scalp peeking through, Penny James, a New York City–based stylist and trichologist (hair and scalp expert), recommends making an appointment with a specialist now. "If you think you are losing hair, you probably are," she told me. "Hair is a barometer that something is going on. Act on it as quickly as you can, since hair loss will often not correct itself." James explains that women's hair loss can be caused by a number of things, including genetics, stress, and medication, and perimenopause is also a biggie. It's worth noting there are other culprits such as a recent bout with food poisoning or adopting a vegan diet. These are correctable, as is switching up a medication that might be the underlying cause. A doctor will help sort it out— make sure to ask that he or she test your thyroid and all your vitamin and mineral levels and check that you are not anemic.

If your hair loss in indeed related to menopause, there are a few things that can be done to slow the process. "Mention it to your ob-gyn," advises James. "She might recommend hormones or supplements." Minoxidil (Rogaine) is the only FDA-approved drug in the United States to combat female pattern baldness. James recommends the 2 percent version. Some dermatologists will prescribe Finasteride, a drug used to shrink an enlarged prostate, for female hair loss, but according to research by the National Institutes of Health the verdict is still out on its effectiveness. *And* the drug can feminize male fetuses, so if there's any chance you might get pregnant, forget it. Five percent Minoxidil is also linked to birth defects. Just because you can buy gallons of something at Costco doesn't mean it's safe.

Consulting an expert will help you feel less vulnerable and find a solution. It may be that your hair seems thin because it's brittle and breaking off, or that you have a vitamin or mineral deficiency, or that your follicles are clogged with city grime. James recommends using a shampoo that's formulated for dry hair or gray hair, which can improve texture and shine (something sulfate- and paraben-free, with balanced pH levels). You don't have to spend a ton of money; according to James, L'Oréal and Procter and Gamble brands spend a lot on research and development, so the appropriate drugstore products are perfectly fine to use.

Personally, I use the special shampoos designed to tackle hair loss (Viviscal seems to help me) and also take a delicious chewy biotin supplement from Whole Foods, and when I'm consistent, they both seem to help.

PUBIC KNOWLEDGE: WAXING, DYING... TRANSPLANTS?!

IT'S NOT JUST MILLENNIALS WHO ARE waxing their cooches to within an inch of their lives. My friend Miranda, married for more than twenty years, has recently started going a little more radical in the waxing arena as a kind of sexy—albeit fucking painful—ritual that adds something new to her two decades of shagging one guy. I do it sometimes too, particularly before a beach vacation. It really does hurt like a motherfucker, and I think I do it for variety more than anything else. I have plenty of girlfriends who sport huge bushes and others who swear by their landing strips. And I've been with men who have a real preference and others who couldn't care less. I also once slept with a guy who was entirely waxed down there, and to me it was a huge turn-off. Talk about regret at the last minute. But the point is, there's no one answer. Do what makes you happy with your pubic hair, for Christ's sake. And be glad you still have it! Eventually, I'm told, it will start to thin out... It's another one of those ironies of age: all the kids are getting waxed to within an inch of their lives, while we are feeling wistful about our balding lady bits.

Speaking of which, have you come in contact with gray pubic hair yet? Your own or someone else's? Holy cow, that can be a shocker. Just writing those three words feels distinctly upsetting. For me it was on a man I was newly sleeping with. Harsh, but less harsh than seeing it on myself, which has thankfully not yet happened. Crotches going gray and bald is very high on my personal list of All Things Unsexy, and yet, it's another reality we must be ready to face. I have one or two friends who occasionally use Betty "bikini" dye, going fuchsia or bright blue down there for fun. It takes forever, apparently (think mascara wand with dye, all down there around your delicate vulva), and I don't have the patience, but again, to each her own! I applaud the ingenuity, the creativity, the fortitude.

I really only mentioned transplants above to make sure you were paying attention. It seems that this *is* done, but it's pretty rare, and mostly to treat a condition called pubic atrichosis (lack of pubic hair), which affects primarily women of Korean and Mongolian descent. Hair follicles are harvested from the back of the scalp using a no-scalpel, no-stitches technique, and then the transplant is performed under anesthesia. Apparently you're good to go for sex in two weeks, and hair growth begins in six to twelve. The wonders of modern medicine.

HOW DOES IT FEEL TO BE JEALOUS OF YOUR DAUGHTER (BABYSITTER, ASSISTANT AT WORK, WAITRESS)?

It feels shitty, but it's not that simple. With my daughters, for example, the jealousy is almost entirely eclipsed by pride, and also a bit of relief. Yes, I feel pangs of envy when I think about all that life they still have in front of them, but if I dig a little deeper, I don't envy them at all. Getting to where I am today wasn't easy (so many breakups, so much loss and therapy, so many tears). When it comes down to it, you really couldn't pay me to go back in time.

The babysitter, the assistant, or the bartender—those women are easier to be jealous of, and it's purely a momentary longing to be that hot and perky again. Remember Snow White's wicked stepmother? She was always "the fairest of them all" to her magic mirror. Until she wasn't. A girlfriend who watched the old Disney version of the story with her children many times never really thought much about the subtext—the wicked stepmother was just some mad, insecure bitch, a sexist stereotype—until her own stepdaughter turned fifteen or sixteen and she found herself feeling she was being eclipsed. All of a sudden, she actually related to the wicked stepmother—she had become that mad insecure bitch!—fading away and watching her stepdaughter bloom. To be so young, with smooth skin and high breasts; to be the one men stare at. What's so great about that anyway? It's all just the superficial ego trip, the validation of being wanted. Come on, ladies: at this point we really can see through all that, can't we? We know what lies on the other side of desire, right? Relationships!

When it comes down to it, would I really want to be twentysomething again? No, definitely not. I like myself, and my life, much more now. I just want those tits; that's all.

OPPP—OTHER PEOPLE'S PRODUCTS AND PHILOSOPHIES

I'VE SHARED WITH YOU WHAT I do in the beauty department, but perhaps more helpful is for you to read what others do, or don't do, if for no other reason than to see that there is never one way, no road map. In a thread inspired by a *Daily Beast* article hilariously titled "I Used to Be Hot, Now I'm Not," Woolfers from all over the world opened up about how far (or not) we go to look good, and how much time and money it really takes:

JENNIFER: I think we know deep down if we are doing things to please others, or to please ourselves. The standard for a fully independent woman shouldn't be a woman who lets herself go. I'll never stop coloring my hair. I do it for me. Does it make me more attractive to men? Probably. If I let it go, I'd look like Paulie Walnuts from the Sopranos.

MICHELLE: I resent the time I spend more than the money. Remember getting out of the shower, throwing on your clothes, and getting out the door? Or washing your face before bed and immediately crawling between the sheets? Now it's body lotion and vitamin C serum and collagen boosters and castor oil on the eyelashes and vitamins and eye cream and lip balm and hand lotion. What used to take me fifteen minutes now takes me thirty—and that's when I don't wear makeup.

HILARY: I spend nothing and do nothing, and it shows. Used to get away with it, not anymore! So, damned if you do, and definitely damned if you don't.

BETTINA: At sixty-two, I find myself venturing out much more frequently without any makeup at all. Because no matter the makeup or occasional filler, I can't make that much of a difference in the way I could when younger…you know, mascara and red lipstick and you're magic. I forget I'm not really pretty anymore. I still feel like it some days when I leave the house, and then I catch sight of myself in a store window…But I can't imagine allowing the gray to come in. Or go to dinner at a nice place without makeup.

LIAT: I wear good-quality lipstick and perfume and factor fifteen face cream, and really that's about it. I color my hair and I'm usually clean.

ALY: I never used any skin care until a few years ago except sunscreen and Aveeno face wash. Now I also use Retin-A.

JUDITH: Botox, fillers, genetics, Vaseline.

What are your rules? What do you consider nonnegotiable, and what will you never do?

THE HIGH COST OF BEAUTY

I'VE REFERRED MORE THAN ONCE to the cost of all this effort, and I'd like to get it out there: there's really no limit to how much money you could invest in your beauty regime. In 2016, the *Wall Street Journal* analyzed the amount four women in their forties spent annually on their looks. They were all white, urban, and relatively affluent. Note that the total outlay included gym memberships and massages, but still, three out of four threw down nearly $20,000 a year, including about $1,500 on face cream alone! And the "frugal" chick spent around $10,000.

Do all those fancy lotions and serums and masks and what have you even make a difference? Have you ever noticed that most men barely even wash their faces, let alone use separate products for eyes, face, neck, and décolletage, and they look just fine? I go to a dermatologist who is probably on the middle of the spectrum—she's happy for me to pay hundreds of dollars on products and procedures, but she doesn't suggest I go whole hog on anything extreme like surgery. My friend Sarah, though, sees a no-nonsense dermatologist for an annual mole check, and this doctor is down-to-earth and fully skeptical. She recommends to Sarah the most basic drugstore products possible, such as Dove soap and Cetaphil. When she got a rash around her eyes from a trendy "organic botanical-based" oil (picked under the full moon, by fairies), the doc told her to moisturize with Vaseline. And when it comes to anti-aging creams (can you guess?), she says, "Retin-A is the only topical product that is effective." This dermatologist's only other nonnegotiable is sunblock. Basically this makes me pretty convinced that I'm a huge sucker. You?

If you simply ask a room of women over fifty what makes them feel young and pretty, you don't actually get a list of products or rules or procedures. This is what I heard:

"Nothing makes me feel younger than my dildo."
"I look my age. I'm just trying not to look like a shitty version of it."
"No sex on top."
"Pink light bulbs."

"Denial."

"I just don't really think about that stuff, and I think insouciance is youthful."

"Loving the shit out of myself (whenever possible)."

"Not trying too hard."

"Telling myself 'Damn, looking good!' as I step out the door often works. As does alcohol."

"Being grateful."

"Regular sex and smiling!"

For those women who have stared themselves down in the mirror and come to terms with their changing looks, not by judging but by accepting, the answer usually is more about attitude than about cosmetics or procedures. I might love a certain cream or procedure, but I'd like to state here for the record that I do think it's all a con, a security blanket more than anything else.

I'M OKAY, YOU'RE OKAY: ACCEPTANCE AND SOLIDARITY

Taking joy in living is a woman's best cosmetic.
—ROSALIND RUSSELL

IF YOU ACCEPT THE IDEA, as I do, that since we were girls our sense of our own value has unfortunately come in a not-insignificant part from our beauty and attractiveness as females, it's a very valid question to wonder what happens to that sense of worth as our looks fade. How do we recalibrate? For some women this transformation (into an "old crone") can be liberating, but for others it can feel scary. My hope is that we start to reshape this narrative and take inspiration from one another. I know so many stunning, vibrant, interesting women with style and grace—from women who dye their pubic hair to women who have waist-length silver manes—and we are all certainly as gorgeous and inspiring as the men we stand next to.

I opened this chapter with a quote from public intellectual Mary Beard, and I'll end it with this inspirational story about her:

Beard is an accomplished genius: a Cambridge professor, the author of several books on ancient Rome, a finalist for a National Book Critics Circle Award, the classics editor of the *Times Literary Supplement*, and a regular contributor to both the *London* and the *New York Review of Books*. She's also, however, a woman (now) in her early sixties, with long gray hair and glasses. When her career in recent years led her to frequent TV appearances, she started getting trolled in the worst way on the Internet. Critics mocked her appearance (calling her "undatable" and flat-out "ugly") with a kind of vitriol that is *never* directed at a man. Beard, who once said, "Barring some sociopaths, probably, there is nobody who doesn't care about their appearance," came right back at her detractors in a series of straightforward and quite funny blog posts, saying, basically, that "this is what fifty-seven looks like." She suggested that all the men (who are so obviously intellectually threatened by her, by the way) who find that hard to swallow should go fuck themselves. Beard is happy with her long gray hair and equally happy to sport chic red shoes. In other words, she's proud of who she is and won't be shamed by her appearance or her age. She became somewhat of a folk hero with her troll slaying, and one of her strongest messages was that feminists could all use a bit more humor around these issues. To which I say, amen, sister!

CHAPTER SIX

(EMOTIONS)

ANXIETY AND DEPRESSION
AND STRESS, OH MY!

*I am here to tell you that one woman, a woman who is
the most undepressed, optimistic, upbeat person I know,
awoke one morning and walked straight into her kitchen and
grabbed a butcher's knife (she is a world-class cook) with the
intent of driving it through her heart. That was menopause.*

*If you take the time to peruse the annals of any
nineteenth-century asylum, as I have, you will discover
that the "cause of admittance" for all women over
forty is listed as* cessation of menses. *Sometimes
I saw the words* change of life, *which sounds like a
euphemism but isn't.*

—MARY RUEFLE, *MY PRIVATE PROPERTY*

IN THE SPRING OF MY forty-fifth year, my maternal grandmother died at the incredible age of 108. (She was technically my step-grandmother, so, no, I didn't win the genetic lottery.) My four teen-age children and I all traveled from our various homes and schools to meet at her funeral in Rochester, New York. At the luncheon fol-lowing the ceremony, as were digging into our baked ziti, one of my daughters, then sixteen, said, "You know, with Grandma dying, I realized for the first time that I'd be more upset if any of my siblings died than if you or Dad died." I put down my fork and drew a breath. Looking over at her across the span of the white tablecloth, I replied, "Well, I'd certainly also prefer that I die before any of you do, so I guess I'm glad you feel that way." She wasn't done, though. She went on: "I mean, you've basically done it all already—you've had a family, had a career, gotten divorced, and remarried. You've traveled. You're essentially done. We still have it all in front of us."

Granted, by this child's logic the beloved woman we were all gathered to celebrate would have been "done" for sixty years between menopause and death (not to mention that my daughter was needling me in that sadistically genius way peculiar to teenagers). Still, her words seemed prophetic.

That spring into summer did indeed prove to be a difficult one. What *was* my value now that my career was in flux, my children didn't need me, and men didn't lust after me as aggressively as they once had? I found myself feeling useless and lost, retreating to my bedroom and closing the curtains a little too often. At this point in my life I was forty-five and nearing an empty nest. I had gotten divorced eight years earlier and at the same time left a two-decade career in book publishing. I had gone back to graduate school and started writing and was trying to carve out a new identity for myself as a writer and consultant, but would it work? I feared that no one would hire me—or care what I had to say. On top of that, I was approaching forty-six, the year my own mother died of breast cancer. Having had a mother die at my age, it seemed all the more possible that I, too, could disappear, and the world would keep on spinning.

I'd describe this period more like hormonally tinged melancholy than clinical depression—and I can say that because I have been clinically depressed at other stages in my life—but it was a dark time. I went back into therapy, started taking Prozac again for a bit, felt less confident and assured than I had in quite a while, and found myself ruminating on my mortality more than might be healthy.

I AM WOMAN, HEAR ME WHIMPER

THE TRUTH IS THAT THE KIND of emotional upheaval I was experiencing is incredibly common among women and not so widely acknowledged. A colleague, Joanna, revealed she felt like her confused misery was dismissed by both her gynecologist and internist, and thus found herself stymied about getting help. Extreme mood swings, loss of sex drive, hot flashes, and weight gain all came on suddenly in her late forties. At her annual physical she described the changes to her doctor, ending with a jokey, "And sometimes I just feel crazy." He looked at her with alarm, so she quickly brushed off her complaints. She was scared...of what? That she would lose her insurance? Be institutionalized? To a certain extent, yes. Mainly, she didn't want to be forever seen by this man of authority as a neurotic, irrational madwoman. She then shared her issues with her female gynecologist, expecting more empathy and help. The response? A patronizing furrowed brow and tutting: "Yes, that happens."

A 2010 paper out of the University of San Francisco describes how much of the research on women's distress at midlife fails to capture the bigger picture of how our profound physical changes are playing out against the elaborate backdrop of our lives. Lead author Marcianna Nosek writes, "A midlife woman's life is complex; she is situated—physically, hormonally, emotionally—in her changing body. She also resides within her social, cultural, and economic environment." Men are allowed, even expected, to have their midlife crises, out of which they (according to myth anyway) will forge renewed meaning and purpose: a hero's journey. Women's midlife, on the other hand, is characterized as a collection of physical symptoms rattling in a closed box that society would prefer not to hear much about anyway. Too often we suffer in silence.

NOT WAVING BUT DROWNING

Nobody heard him, the dead man,
But still he lay moaning:
I was much further out than you thought
And not waving but drowning.

Poor chap, he always loved larking
And now he's dead
It must have been too cold for him his heart gave way,
They said.

Oh, no no no, it was too cold always
(Still the dead one lay moaning)
I was much too far out all my life
And not waving but drowning.
—STEVIE SMITH

NOT WAVING, OR DROWNING, OR EVEN SLEEPING

SO MANY OF US ARE HAVING trouble sleeping, and not just because of hot flashes, but because of an anxiety that creeps in like a malicious intruder in the middle of the night. Or we have late-afternoon slumps, or we despise our families come the weekend. Women don't talk about it much because we're afraid of the social stigma, of being seen as weak, which is ridiculous given the staggering numbers of women affected. The Mayo Clinic reports that twice as many women as men experience depression; that's about 12 million American women in any given year. Rates of anxiety and sleeplessness are also higher for women than for men, according to the World Health Organization.

There has been much research that suggests that women's hormonal fluctuations are linked to an increase in mood disorders and depression, including work by the Penn Ovarian Aging Study and the Harvard Study of Moods and Cycles. As menopause approaches, depression and anxiety may take hold of women who never experienced these issues before, and it may well be worse for those who have. The exact mechanisms are still not fully understood. As USF lead author Nosek points out, you need to look at the totality of a woman's life to understand why she might be experiencing emotional distress. Insomnia, transitions with partners or children, physical aging, hormones—it's a tangle of factors that impact us.

Here are some of the things that stress me out pretty much all the time, from the mundane to the existential:

- So much paperwork: bills to pay, mail to read, emails to answer, insurance forms to fill out, and trains or planes or buses to book.

- So much laundry to do. And then the washer breaks. And there's always another light bulb to replace.

- Keeping the house clean and organized. How is it that closets magically repopulate with crap and socks *always* get lost?

- Taking the dog to the vet. Feeding the dog. Walking the dog.

- Grocery shopping always, and it's so boring. I remember my mother complaining that she was out of ideas for meal planning, and, God, yes, me too.

- All of the above, over and over again; it never ends. Until it truly ends.

- How will we pay for everything endlessly? What if we run out of money, can't get decently paid jobs?

- Staying on top of my medical needs and the medical needs of my four children. How do other people manage to keep everyone's teeth cleaned and hair cut? It seems like it would be very easy to forget to fill a tooth or get a mammogram or make sure child number four gets that strange mole checked.

■ Little kids, little problems; big kids, big problems. Thinking about the genuine risks our teens and twentysomethings are taking or the problems they are facing can be the stuff of nightmares.

■ The world can be a horrible place; people starving, bombs falling, corrupt politicians, global warming, plastic bottles choking the oceans, lousy health care access, lousy public education, potholes! Why did I bring children into this world in the first place?

■ Car accidents, cancer, strokes, rapes, murder—there are so many awful things that can and do happen to people every day. How do I even get up in the morning?

■ What am I forgetting? Have I answered all my emails? Life is so endlessly 24/7 these days that it just feels impossible to ever rest.

■ Am I part of the problem or part of the solution? Have I made any sort of difference in the world? And does it even matter?

My friend Wendy, who is in her late fifties, often calls me when she is distressed. More than once during these teary phone calls, she has brought up a shared memory of an afternoon, almost twenty years ago, when our eldest children were toddlers. Wendy and I had met and become friends because the girls were in preschool together, and on the summer day in question we had both taken the Friday afternoon off, I from my job in publishing, she from her job in public relations. At the time I belonged to a gym in Manhattan's West Village, and this gym had a pool on the roof. We brought the girls and sat out on the deck by the water, sunning and talking and watching them splash on the steps. I was wearing a yellow bikini and Wendy wore a huge glamorous black hat. I remember this day too, but for Wendy it seems to have stuck in her mind as an emblem of a time when things were easier, when our lives had so much promise. She asks me, "Why can't we have days like that anymore?" And I do know what she means. Why does it feel like everything has sped up so much? Is it because we have a smaller percentage of our lives left? It's not that we don't have good times anymore, but it often feels to me like things get harder as we get older, not easier. The responsibilities grow; the worries are ever present. Sometimes this strikes me as unfair; I've worked so hard, tried so hard; can't I get a break? What happened to "older and wiser" or the concept of the golden years? I suspect that might all be crap.

WHY ARE WE SO DEPRESSED?

Life is an unstable system in which balance
is continually lost and continually recovered.
—SIMONE DE BEAUVOIR, *THE COMING OF AGE*

YES, WE DO GET DOWN. The two-to-one ratio of depression in women versus men persists across racial, ethnic, and economic divides and is found in most countries around the world. I think if you add to the pressures of regular life the features that are particular to life over forty for women—hormonal fluctuations, lack of sleep, hot flashes, teenagers, aging parents, sagging bodies, wrinkles, chin hairs, achy knees, financial worries, looming retirement—you inevitably get a rocky stew of emotional challenges. Here are the greatest hits for ladies in our cohort, and I'd be very surprised if you don't see yourself somewhere in here:

■ **Perimenopause and menopause.** Yes, if you didn't already get this memo, women are at increased risk for depression during perimenopause—in fact, one of the documented symptoms of perimenopause is "impending sense of doom," which makes me laugh even though it's so dark.

■ **Health problems.** You've heard me talk about my tennis elbow. For more than a year it ached every time I picked up a jar of peanut butter, making me feel like a pathetic old lady, and now that it's gone I have a shoulder problem. Putting on a jacket hurts. A bunch of my friends have a slew of new aches and pains, from foot and knee issues to lower back pain, and it can be a serious bummer to not be as nimble as we once were, as well as hurting basically all the time. Not to mention much worse chronic illness or disability: cancer, stroke, cardiac disease, high cholesterol, diabetes, the list goes on. It probably goes without saying that physical infirmity can lead to depression.

■ **Fixating on and rehashing negative feelings.** Women tend to sit in our own crap more than men do. We're more likely to cry to relieve emotional tension, to try to figure out why we're depressed, and to talk to our friends about our unhappiness. But rumination has been found to maintain depression and even make it worse! According to a meta-analysis by neuroscience and psychology researchers at the University of Colorado, women's brooding and reflection have a direct link to our higher levels of misery. Men, on the other hand, are more inclined to distract themselves when they are depressed. Unlike rumination, distraction can reduce depression. Maybe this is a place where we should take the lead from dudes. In an interview, my therapist, Dr. Debbie Magids, told me, "We have a thread in our minds about what's wrong with us. We need to shift that to what's great about us. What good are we doing in the world?"

Overwhelming stress. Whether it comes from work, school, or home, marriage problems, death of a loved one, teenagers sending us over the edge, elderly parents needing care, or money issues, some studies show that women are more likely than men to develop depression from stress. On top of working outside of the home, we clock twice as much time as our male partners doing housework and being caregivers. We also deal with workplace discrimination and everyday sexism. On top of this, according to the National Institute of Mental Health, we produce more stress hormones than men do, and the female sex hormone progesterone prevents the stress hormone system from turning itself off as it does in men. I feel it all the time; do you? Our bodies conspire against us here, yet again...

■ **Body image issues.** Before adolescence, boys and girls experience mood disorders at about the same rate. After puberty, girls are twice as likely to suffer from depression or anxiety as boys. One related factor is poor body image and its impact on self-esteem. Hideously, these issues plague us throughout our adult lives. According to a study published by the *Journal of Health Psychology*, women who are more concerned about their physical appearance are more likely to feel negative about menopause. *And* women who feel negative about menopause are more likely to experience mood disorders and health problems during menopause. Um…? This feels very no-win to me.

■ **Thyroid issues.** Women also have a higher incidence of thyroid problems than men, and hypothyroidism can cause depression, so always ask about your thyroid during your annual physical. And it should go without saying: always get an annual physical.

SO WHAT TO DO ABOUT IT? PROZAC (AND XANAX AND VALIUM) NATION

Like a lot of people, I had a resistance [to taking anti-depressants], thinking that emotional or mental problems are things that you can deal with other than through medication. I also didn't want anything to affect me mentally. But what a difference! And I thought, "Boy, what a different childhood I might have had had my mother taken antidepressants."

—AMY TAN, *TIME*, MARCH 5, 2001

MORE THAN 50 PERCENT OF WOMEN who responded to a recent survey by the nonprofit Mental Health America said they thought that depression was a normal part of aging and menopause and doesn't warrant treatment. That just makes me really sad. Depression should be acknowledged and dealt with. It may not require medication, but how about talk therapy, more sleep, yoga, herbal tea…something! It's important to be real with yourself, to take stock, and to spend some time soul searching.

Debbie Magids advises her clients not to be afraid of the sadness, emptiness, or loss that can accompany all the transitions women go through at midlife. "Feel your loss so you can feel what you gain on the other side." Try to figure out if your distress about the physiological symptoms of menopause might be signaling that another area of your life, such as your relationship or career, isn't working.

And then there are drugs.

I went on Prozac in my late twenties—my mother had died, I had an absentee father, my childhood pain was huge and crippling—and stayed on it for more than ten years. The way I always described being on an antidepressant to friends was that it just ever so subtly took the edge off. I never felt medicated or numb, but I did feel just slightly calmer, more able to deal with life, and less prone to paralyzing sadness. I've heard others say the right medication made them feel like themselves again. In my thirties, as my first marriage deteriorated, I associated the Prozac with mollifying me in an unhappy union, so when I left the relationship I also ditched the Prozac. During that period I tried Klonopin and Lexapro, and neither worked for me, but during the initial weeks of our separation I was completely numbed up on Ativan. Back to Prozac for another few years (lesson: when you find an antidepressant that works for you, stick with it), and these days, after paying off a college degree's worth of therapy bills, I'm medication-free, but I always keep a prescription of Xanax on hand for emergencies. Half a Xanax is a lifesaver in so many situations—a bad election outcome, a hideous fight with my husband, a sleepless night when I can't reach one of my children—and I'm grateful that these drugs exist.

When I think back to my childhood, watching my mother struggle with a level of anger and depression that often left her closeted in her room for days at a time (wow, it *just* occurred to me that I get that habit from her! bingo!), I, too, can only imagine how my (and her) experience might have been different if she had sought the help of a good psychiatrist and therapist. I know women who say they lost precious years to anxiety or depression when they could have been living more fully and with more joy had they spoken up to their doctor. Drugs are not a magic cure-all, but they can reinforce the basic functionality that gets you out of bed, interacting with people, and getting stuff done. For some, the appropriate antidepressant can literally be a lifesaver.

A word on addiction: I have many other character flaws and biological weaknesses, but addiction does not appear to be one of them. I quit smoking cigarettes on a dime in my twenties; I can easily stop drinking alcohol for months if I want to eat healthier or lose weight. This isn't a boast. I mention it because it's easy for me to be a fan of antidepressants and antianxiety medication when I know the like-lihood that I will develop a dependence on them is low. For others that's not the case. Drugs used to treat anxiety disorders, especially benzodiazepines such as Xanax, Valium, and Klonopin, are addic-tive and definitely have the potential for abuse. They should be pre-scribed with caution and oversight, especially to those with a history of alcohol or substance abuse. When I get my prescription, my doc-tor stingily hands out twenty pills. My friend Kenny has some quack doctor who gives him 120 pills at a time! *Not safe!* Be careful, please: any medication should be used correctly and under the care of a reputable, qualified physician.

While I may be a proponent of finding the right meds as neces-sary, when a good friend in crisis asked me to reach out to the Woolf-ers for group support, *not a single one* brought up pharmaceuticals. Friendship and self-care were their first line of defense against the blues.

> What are your best tips for comfort, diversion, dis-traction, and healing in times of extreme personal distress? A dear girlfriend is going through a bad breakup (divorced, kids grown). She's the type who doesn't like being alone, is always on to the next man (which I relate to big-time), and I can feel her pain of sitting with this moment and want to help. I suggested picking up a new hobby (French lessons, anyone?) and rattled off my current fave binge shows. Any ideas from the hive?

EMILY: I could not have gotten through hard times without my women friends. And I have to say that being partnerless right now is really okay because of them. They are my anchor, my sounding board, and thank goodness, my social life. #howdomensurvive?

ANDREA: First and foremost leaning in to your friends definitely. Self-care (yoga, meditation, massage, reflection). Diving into the creative self-expressive arts, journaling, photography, dance, movement. And if she's able, taking an "upside down trip," meaning something out of the ordinary.

DENA: How about a dog? My dog, Julie, saved me during my divorce. A million walks, a million hours of training, all helped me manage my pain. And by the time the divorce storm passed, I ended up with the most well-behaved dog in the world.

LAURA: Being comfortable with being uncomfortable is really important.

DEIRDRE: Exercise. Weight lifting to feel strong, boudoir or pole dancing to feel sexy.

SHELAGH: Art. Literature. Nature. And I will add my own mother's advice: "When you feel sorry for yourself, help someone else."

And from a Woolfer who is also a therapist, Susan Epstein:

> Avoid should and experiment with rhythm. Let yourself be in between, emotionally expressive, uncertain. Write stories about your choices with different endings. Do some finger painting or make a collage without having an agenda or caring what it will look like when you are done. Unleash your unconscious by doing things that are immersive: go swimming, dance at a club by yourself, "call in sick" (if you have that kind of life/job/situation), and see a movie in the middle of the day. Mix it up! Listen to your gut.

HOW BAD DO I HAVE IT?

Come, pain, feed on me. Bury your fangs in my flesh.
Tear me asunder. I sob, I sob.
—VIRGINIA WOOLF, *THE WAVES*

DEPRESSION IS NEVER one size fits all. It can be mild or severe, can last for a few days, a few years, or a lifetime. Everyone has feelings of sadness and loss that eventually fade. Clinical depression, on the other hand, is a medical condition that interferes with your daily life and can't be shaken off by "thinking positive," "counting your blessings," or any other pep talk offered by well-meaning but ultimately not-very-helpful people around you. Basically, if you have been experiencing any of the following symptoms for more than two weeks, you should see your doctor (the National Institute of Mental Health backs me up on this):

- Persistent sad, anxious, or "empty" mood
- Feelings of hopelessness or pessimism
- Irritability
- Feelings of guilt, worthlessness, or helplessness
- Decreased energy or fatigue
- Difficulty sleeping, early-morning awakening, or oversleeping
- Loss of interest or pleasure in hobbies and activities
- Moving or talking more slowly
- Feeling restless or having trouble sitting still
- Difficulty concentrating, remembering, or making decisions
- Appetite and/or weight changes
- Thoughts of death or suicide, or suicide attempts
- Aches or pains, headaches, cramps, or digestive problems without a clear physical cause and/or that do not ease even with treatment

SOURCE: NATIONAL INSTITUTE OF MENTAL HEALTH (NIMH)

Also, did you know that the way men and women experience depression is often radically different? I find this fascinating and relevant: I live with both a husband and a son. It's interesting to me to think about the ways we process and express our sadness differently, and if we can't understand each other, we're pretty stuck. Not only are we more prone to depression than the men in our lives, but the causes of our sadness and even the patterns of our symptoms are generally quite different.

For example, seasonal affective disorder—depression in the winter months due to lower levels of sunlight—is more common in women than in men. Women are also more likely to experience the symptoms of atypical depression.

NOT NORMAL? WHAT IS ATYPICAL DEPRESSION?

Rather than sleeping less, eating less, and losing weight, the opposite happens: sleeping excessively, eating more (especially carbohydrates), and gaining weight. Sound familiar? Feelings of guilt associated with depression are also more prevalent and pronounced in women than in men.

DIFFERENCES BETWEEN MALE AND FEMALE DEPRESSION	
WOMEN TEND TO:	MEN TEND TO:
Blame themselves	Blame others
Feel sad, apathetic, and worthless	Feel angry, irritable, and ego inflated
Feel anxious and scared	Feel suspicious and guarded
Avoid conflicts at all costs	Create conflicts
Feel slowed down and nervous	Feel restless and agitated
Have trouble setting boundaries	Need to feel in control at all costs
Find it easy to talk about self-doubt and despair	Find it "weak" to admit self-doubt or despair
Use food, friends, and "love" to self-medicate	Use alcohol, TV, sports, and sex to self-medicate

ADAPTED FROM: *MALE MENOPAUSE* BY JED DIAMOND

Does this ring a bell? It really does for me, and it helps me have a little more empathy for all of us, both men and women, as we navigate through our many struggles.

AM I REALLY MY MOTHER? AND OTHER QUESTIONS TO ASK YOUR THERAPIST

*Owning our story can be hard but not nearly
as difficult as spending our lives running from it.*
—BRENÉ BROWN

IN MY YOUNGER YEARS, from twenty to my midthirties, I saw quite a few therapists who didn't help much. There was a string (at least three) of kindly middle-aged women with frizzy hair and potted plants (kind of like me now) who nodded and sympathized, but I don't remember ever feeling that epiphanic click of "Yes! I get it! That's why I do/feel/say that." Going to therapy with the wrong person can be really discouraging and can also feel like an enormous waste of money. But trust me, when you connect with the right person, it's like night and day.

When I was thirty-seven, I left the father of my four children, a man I'd been with for sixteen mostly unhappy years. I had felt lonely and ignored, was deeply depressed, and at the very end was having an affair with my yoga teacher. It was awful. And to the confusion of everyone around me, who saw our separation as me leaving him, I was also furious, almost perpetually enraged. I was terrified to upend my life and traumatize my children, but I had reached a point where I really felt like I'd die if I stayed. All the rage and grief went back to my childhood (no surprise there, right?), but I hadn't been able untangle all the issues and connections. At the time, I was not in therapy, but I was getting Prozac from a psychopharmacologist who one day said to me, "You know, I really think you need to see someone." He gave me the card of a woman named Dr. Debbie Magids, and I carried that card around in my purse for at least a month. I was so sick of seeing therapists who didn't help me, and my story felt so big and ugly; the idea of regurgitating it for yet another person made me want to crawl into a cave. But I was also cursing like a sailor on steroids, screaming, crying, and behaving in ways that were pretty scary, so I finally called and went to see her.

Debbie virtually saved my life. She's my age, and from Long Island, with long blown-out hair and legs that never end. For whatever reason (she's a genius? I was ready? we just click?), pretty much every single session with Debbie moves me to a different place. I saw her three times a week for nearly two years, then went down to twice a week, then once, and then one day, around the six-year mark, she said to me, "You know, as much as I love you, I need to tell you that you don't need to be here anymore." Whoa. At that point I was so attached, the idea of leaving was actually traumatizing in itself. She kindly added, "There's always more to work on, and you can come back to me for tune-ups whenever you want, but you need to know that you are in good shape and you really don't need me." I spent another six or nine months hanging on, and then it started to dawn on me that I might like that time back and could use the money for other things. I started to like the idea of leaving. So I did. But we remain close, and I do go back for tune-ups, sometimes just for a session or two, and sometimes I go back for months at a time. And the secret truth? I consider her my best friend. The person who knows me best and whom I trust implicitly, and whom I always know will help me. Even though I pay her. And I know she loves me too.

It's amazing to me when people are resistant to therapy. Some of the people I love most in the world are classic examples. They know dozens of people who see therapists; they know I worship mine. And yet, when I suggest they seek help by talking to someone, I'm met with hostility and resistance. Are they afraid of what they may need to face? Do they really have no time for self-care? Or are they ashamed, or just bored by the prospect of self-examination? Whatever the case, it bums me out. I can think of almost no greater gift you can give yourself than exploring who you are with an objective, educated outsider, someone who doesn't judge or have an investment in what you do when and to whom.

My friend Julie says she avoids therapy just because it's a lot of hard work. "Going in once a week and ripping a Band-Aid off the wounds I work so hard to keep under wraps is not exactly appealing, especially when I'm trying to 'keep it together' in other areas of my life. I obviously recognize that that's self-defeating, but it's a pretty good rationalization too. Ha." She's not alone. Another friend, Sadie, says, "I personally don't feel comfortable talking to a 'stranger.' I'd rather speak to my friends. I feel weird about paying to talk to someone, but I recognize it's a great help to many and perhaps would be for me." So there are all sorts of thoughts on this front, but at the very least, I encourage you to consider it. Look what our friend from *Scandal* says on the subject:

> I say that publicly because I think it's really import-
> ant to take the stigma away from mental health...My
> brain and my heart are really important to me. I don't

know why I wouldn't seek help to have those things be as healthy as my teeth. I go to the dentist. So why wouldn't I go to a shrink?

—KERRY WASHINGTON, *GLAMOUR*, APRIL 2015

Who among us doesn't think that Olivia Pope's advice is worth following?

Finding a great therapist who also takes insurance is a big deal, I'll grant you. According to a 2016 article in the *Wall Street Journal*, more than half of all counties in the United States have no practicing psychiatrists, psychologists, or social workers. Asking trusted friends and your physician for referrals is a first step. The *Psychology Today* website also has a therapy directory where you can enter your zip code to find nearby therapists and see whether or not they take insurance or offer a sliding-scale fee. Your state Medicaid office can provide information on practitioners who accept Medicaid.

STUCK IN THE MIDDLE OF THE SANDWICH GENERATION WITHOUT ANY CONDIMENTS

TAKING CARE OF AGING PARENTS and hostile teenagers just as your looks are fading, your body hurts in weird places for no reason, and you can no longer get an uninterrupted night of sleep. Sounds great, right? My own parents are dead, and so are my in-laws, and as much as we miss them, I've thought more than once (guiltily) that I'm lucky in that way. I'm really not sure how I could have handled nursing home and college applications at the same time.

According to the Pew Research Center, nearly half of adults in their forties and fifties have a parent aged sixty-five or older and are either raising a young child or financially supporting a grown child at the same time. It's not surprising that this takes a financial toll: for people in the "sandwich generation," 30 percent say they have enough money to meet their basic expenses with a little left over for extras. Another 30 percent say they are only able to pay for their essentials, and 11 percent don't have enough to cover even the basics.

There's a massive emotional toll as well, especially for women. According to the Family Caregiver Alliance as many as 75 percent of family members taking care of an elderly parent are women, regardless of employment or parenting status or other responsibilities. My friend Marnie had her daughter in her early forties. In her midfifties, at the same time she was experiencing middle-of-the-night sweat baths coupled with labor pain–like gushing periods, her daughter started her period. As with many younger teens, it came with crazy mood swings and lots of stained sheets and underwear for Mom to clean up. Meanwhile, her seventy-five-year-old father got dementia and started pooping his pants like an infant, often in her car, on the way to one of the many doctor's appointments he had each month. Did I mention that her company was going through round after round of layoffs, so while she was coping with her family challenges, she also faced the threat of losing their primary income and health insurance?

The University of Michigan Depression Center estimates that

between 20 and 50 percent of people caring for their parents suffer from depression—the number skews highest for women. As caregivers, women often neglect their own needs, which can lead to the risk of developing chronic diseases such as high blood pressure and cardiovascular problems. There can be conflicts in marriages and with other family members. Sadly, in our fragmented society, there isn't much of a safety net for unpaid caregivers of any kind. It does take a village, one that we don't have.

What you can do is recognize when you are overwhelmed, determine if there's anyone else who can pitch in, take time for yourself, and set boundaries. A cousin's eighty-year-old father was leaving as many as twenty messages an hour on her home answering machine, so she cut off her landline; her postcollege son was living in his old bedroom while he searched for a job but was mainly watching movies and playing video games, and she cut off his Internet. Take charge; do what you need to do to take care of yourself. When my kids were little, I went by the maxim "If I'm not taking care of myself, I can't take care of them." The same thing applies when we are getting it on both ends.

DIVORCE ENVY

*I really don't advise a woman who wants to have
things her own way to get married.*
—VIRGINIA WOOLF

THE LONG MARRIED AMONG US sometimes suffer from a little divorce envy. Being with the same partner forever has definite high points (the deep intimacy, the family all together), but it can also be boring as hell sometimes. For a lot of women I know, trying to spice up sex after twenty-five years is a real challenge, and there's also just that what-if feeling. What if I never experience anything else again? What if he really is the last man I'll ever kiss? Can I live with that? No one answer is the same, of course, but it's worth looking at. The fact is, getting older comes with lots of wistful contemplation...

My friend Eliza told me this story: "I had only been married a few years when I heard an older woman friend grumble about her husband: 'I'm having a Merry Widow fantasy.' Huh? It would take a few more years before I really understood the sentiment and found myself imagining what my life would be like if my husband were dead (a gentle, peaceful death, nothing too gruesome so as not to upset the children). Another daydream was getting a divorce, selling my over-stuffed house, moving into a spic-and-span little apartment, and furnishing it in single a day with a call to West Elm."

A good friend of mine, Shelly, married an older divorced guy when she was in her thirties. He already had a daughter and then together they had two more. Fast-forward twenty-five years and her husband, John, is nearing seventy, alcoholic, and severely depressed. And has been for many years. Life is not great, but they bumble along together, out of comfort, and loyalty, and a lot of inertia. Shelly, meanwhile, is a vibrant fifty-four. She started her own PR business a few years ago and is killing it. She travels a lot for work and meets interesting people, and her daughters are launched, and she comes home to this extremely sad sack of a man. I have divorce envy *for* her. Is that a terrible thing to admit? I want her to be happy, to feel appreciated, to have a few more grand adventures before she gets old and dies. A part of her feels the same way, but of course she feels guilty about it. She may one day leave; time will tell.

On the other end of the spectrum, four years ago I scraped my girlfriend Jenn off the pavement after *her* husband of twenty-five years left her for another woman. She got on with her life like a trouper, moving house, taking care of the kids he didn't seem to have much time for anymore, working, saving money for enriching, healthy vacations like yoga retreats and walking in France, but she was in deep, deep mourning. She believed she would be single forever and said she was sure her vagina would simply close up shop. And then she met an attractive, sweet guy. After spending her whole adult life with the same man, she got the opportunity to have a wild, heart-pounding crush and intense, passionate sex. Since she had done so much work building a solid new life for herself, she didn't necessarily want to partner up again. Her boyfriend was just the cherry on top.

On the other side of divorce envy, of course, is the very real relationship envy that we can all imagine if we aren't living it. It can be a very nice and comfy and safe feeling to be in a relationship. I love waking up next to my husband every day. I love his heft and gruffness and maleness. Even when he's driving me completely crazy, there's often no one else I'd rather be with, and that's a huge gift. Not easy to find. (Also not easy to maintain, but I remind myself how hard it is to find and I keep working on it!) The years between my two marriages were fun in certain ways, but the angst of trying to find someone to love was real and lonely and had me pretty blue at times.

DEATH HAPPENS: OUR PARENTS, OUR PARTNERS, OUR FRIENDS, OUR OWN

THEN THERE'S THE FACT THAT our friends are actually starting to get sick and die. And this is a trend that will not be reversing itself.

Inevitable, impending death, our own and the deaths of those we love, is a huge downer. And I'm not joking. Remember my daughter's snarky comments after my grandmother's funeral about how I had hit my sell-by date and was thus virtually useless? I've just passed the relatively early age when my mother died, and none of us will ever be any younger than we are today. Every cough, lump, strange spot on my skin: these could all be cancer one day. Or I could have a stroke or get hit by a car. On an autumn day, I'll find myself looking at bare trees in the park and wondering, at this point on the age continuum, am I living or dying? And when I bought a pair of really sturdy winter boots recently, I thought, "Could this be the last pair of sturdy boots I'll ever buy?" I catch myself in these maudlin thoughts and laugh, but they are actually true. Death is everywhere, and this is just the reality, always, for all of us. It's something we shy away from discussing in our youth-obsessed culture, but I think there's enormous value in looking at it head-on. As Irvin Yalom writes in his brave book, *Staring at the Sun*:

> Death…is always with us, scratching at some inner door, whirring softly, barely audibly, just under the membrane of consciousness. Hidden and disguised,

leaking out in a variety of symptoms, it is the well-spring of many of our worries, stresses, and conflicts.

I feel strongly...that confronting death allows us, not to open some noisome Pandora's box, but to re-enter life in a richer, more compassionate manner.

Thinking about our inevitable demise can give meaning to the everyday. It's simplistic, but so true: how better to appreciate today than to contemplate it being your last? The psychologist and Buddhist meditation teacher Tara Brach has an exercise she totes out frequently: ask yourself what you would do if you had one year to live. What about a month, a week, a day? Consider spending a few minutes answering these questions and see what comes up. It's a step toward figuring out what is truly important to you and worth spending (precious) time on. As my therapist Debbie Magids said to me, "If not now, when?"

I'm afraid of entering a phase of my life where the deaths of friends and loved ones will become routine, but if I'm lucky enough to live a long life, that's what will happen. So these are hard truths we need to contemplate, and they speak to the crux of all of life's mystery. Why are we here? What does it all mean? How do I manage the pain of loss and suffering?

HOW TO EMBRACE YOUR INNER BITCH (AND NOT WIND UP ALONE, DEAD, AND HALF-EATEN BY CATS)

ONE STEREOTYPE OF OLDER WOMEN, or really just grown women, is the hard and shrill biddy, the "nasty woman" of the 2016 election cycle. She's a woman who speaks her mind and complains and demands. Who says what she thinks in a bitchy, sometimes condescending way because she's sick of having to tiptoe around an issue. She doesn't want to "be nice"; she wants to get shit done. The pushy woman. The one with the RBF (resting bitch face) who does not "smile" on command. I think you may know her. Sometimes we're demanding. Sometimes we're fucking angry. Is this really a problem?

I myself cried when I got angry, then became unable to explain why I was angry in the first place. Later I would discover this was endemic among female human beings. Anger is supposed to be "unfeminine," so we suppress it—until it overflows.

I could see that not speaking up made my mother feel worse. This was my first hint of the truism that depression is anger turned inward; thus women are twice as likely to be depressed.

—GLORIA STEINEM, *MY LIFE ON THE ROAD*

Personally, expressing anger has never been hard for me. On the contrary, I've had to work hard to understand it (so often anger covers up fear or pain) and learn how to deploy it sensibly and when appropriate. Inappropriate anger is pretty easy to recognize: yelling at the checkout guy when he's too slow; screaming at someone who meant well but maybe came up short; cutting people off in traffic just because you can. These behaviors are not so nice. Take a deep breath.

But what is appropriate anger? Maybe when one of your children is being misunderstood or mistreated by a teacher. That might be a moment to stand up and raise your voice. Or when your partner is dismissive for the tenth time about something you really care about and you want to be heard. When you get whipped into a fury over some injustice in the world. Or even when you come home after a long day and the kids haven't done the dishes or their homework and they promised they would.

So many women suffer from an inability to confront a problem directly without getting upset, feeling vulnerable, or feeling unentitled to complain. It's a delicate balance. There's a line between managing the frustrations of daily life with composure and feeling like you are being mistreated or taken advantage of. There's no good reason to be a doormat, and the idea of being "ladylike" in the face of mean, abusive, or exploitative behavior is garbage in my book. The answer lies in being yourself. Listen to your truth. Pay attention to what you (or those you are fighting for) need, and know you deserve to get it. You might even be surprised to find that people listen and respond! If you can harness your inner bitch and use her for good, maybe the anger won't spill over in the wrong places.

And besides, you're not being a bitch if you're asserting your-self and drawing a line. That's just you being you. And we love you for it.

SUNDAY WITH THE FAMILY MALAISE

Have you ever looked up from your coffee and the paper on a Sunday morning and felt like you wanted to murder each and every member of your family? This seems to be fairly common for women in the throes of perimenopause. My friend Kristen once said, "Monday is a day of recovery." To borrow a phrase from writer Sandra Tsing Loh, as we get older, our "estrogen cloud"—that vapor that compelled us to cookie-cutter sandwiches into "fun" shapes for our finicky child, to take care of neglected fish and hamsters and turtles, to fold everybody's underwear—drifts away, and we're left feeling really fucking sick and tired of managing everyone's schedule and junk and moods.

My friend Leslie and her twentysomething daughter and said daughter's boyfriend all live in Boston. Wednesday or Thursday each week Leslie gets a bubbly text: *"Hi Mom! When are we seeing you this weekend? How about we come over for Sunday brunch? Emoji emoji emoji."* Every single time Leslie flinches and wonders if she can just pretend she didn't see it. Sunday brunch means more cooking, more dishes (or more money spent on a restaurant), and less opportunity to sleep, read, take a walk, go to a museum, or do yoga or any of the other activities she does to stay sane before another week rolls around. She loves her kids like a mama bear, but she also cherishes her downtime. There's nothing wrong with that, and it's up to us to draw the lines.

DIGGING YOUR WAY OUT OF THE DUMPS

IF YOU AREN'T CLINICALLY DEPRESSED or suffering from an anxiety disorder or another condition that warrants treatment, there are so many ways to shake off the blues. Keep in mind that, as my therapist, Debbie, says, "There's no woman on the planet who feels good all the time, but every day is a new day and a chance to reset and try again."

DO: EXERCISE. EVERY. SINGLE. DAY.

Tons of studies show that moving your ass for thirty minutes every day makes you feel better. Get up, get out! I can't say I achieve this, but I do try. And I need to constantly switch up my routine, otherwise, I get bored. I've been through many exercise phases: yoga, Pilates, Spinning, Zumba, tennis, personal trainers, and so on, and usually after a year or two I move on to the next thing.

I hate running, truly detest the huffing and puffing, and have never once come close to a runner's high, but this year, at age forty-seven, I committed to running my first 5K with a bunch of girlfriends. I used an app called Couch to 5K (there are many others) that employs a progressive walk-run-jog-walk scenario that gradually gets you up to running the full 3.2 miles over many weeks. It was a great challenge, and even though it was sometimes torture, I did start to feel pretty good (a teensy bit thinner and so psyched to refer to myself as a "runner" for the first time in my life) as I approached the race. The race itself—on a gorgeous, glorious November day in Central Park with a few other Woolfers—was a complete revelation. It was so much fun, I signed up for a four-mile "Jingle Jog" race the following month! My point: try new things. Challenge yourself. Make it something fun and hard, and you'll really feel proud of yourself when you see improvement. Self-pride is a big mood booster.

DO: GET SHIT DONE

I'm a huge to-do lister. Nothing makes me happier (well, okay, sex and a new pair of shoes might make me happier, but hopefully you get the point) than drafting a long, stressed-out to-do list on a Monday morning and then making calls and sending emails and going places in my car, and one by one, striking the things off the list. Being proactive, as opposed to passive and whiny, can make you the Wonder Woman of your own crisis.

DON'T: GO INTO HIDING

My tendency, as I've said, is to take to my bed for hours at a time, but never days. I have some good friends, though, who hibernate when they are depressed. They don't answer their phones, or they hide in their cubicles at work or call in sick. In fact, I always know my bestie Samantha is depressed when I don't hear from her for more than five days. I get it. When I feel bluesy or sorry for myself, I generally don't want to admit it. I'm often embarrassed by my fragility, and I feel guilty for potentially dragging others down with me. In that state, I believe I should be able to fix myself, like, "My feelings are pathetic, I'm a loser, blah, blah, blah." This is crazy talk. *Everyone struggles*, no matter how perfect his or her life might seem from the outside, and *everyone needs help sometimes.* Don't be ashamed, and know when to ask for help.

It's vitally important to know *whom* you can go to. *Before* there's a crisis, identify who in your circle is actually helpful. Who comforts you? Who knows the exact right thing to say? Who provides a judgment-free safe space and can be completely trusted with your woes?

When I was younger, there were always one or two best friends I'd call on with every slight. While I still love my circle of girlfriends, and do know I can rely on them, I have to admit that my number one go-to person has become my therapist. As I get older I find myself less inclined to wallow (in part, I feel like I have less time), and Debbie cuts straight to the heart of whatever is bringing me down. She helps me sort out how much of a problem is in my own head, how much is a reality that I have to figure out how to deal with, and how much might be someone else's crap.

Find people you can confide in and keep them close.

DO: EAT HEALTHY FOOD INSTEAD OF THE GARBAGE YOU WANT TO EAT

Yes, another tip that is easier said than done, and easier for some than for others. What I've found as I get older is that sugar, gluten, and alcohol make me feel like absolute trash. I notice the effects right away. Good pizza and wine have been my favorite things for years, but I've pretty much cut both out of my diet to simply feel like a human with a life worth living. It's the same with sugar. I cave sometimes—love chocolate sorbet, love the occasional croissant with butter and jam—but for the most part it's honestly not worth it anymore. I notice it right away: if I have one cookie, I want more. In fact, any bread or baked goods or dessert or wine makes me crave more, and soon I'm bloated and cranky and awake at four a.m. sweating buckets. Who needs it? And going without means I'm a teensy bit skinnier too, and that's a mood and confidence booster. So suddenly, right around age forty-six, certain foods became a trade-off that no longer made sense to me.

Women tend to crave carbs when they are down, and scientists speculate that that's due to a dip in serotonin. You might get a quick boost from sugar or foods that are made from refined flour products, but it doesn't last. My go-to snacks are carrots and celery with hummus, olives, dates dipped in almond butter, and rolled-up slices of salami and turkey. If I do have a drink (which has become less and less frequent), I have tequila (or any distilled liquor) with club soda and fresh lime instead of wine or a sugary cocktail. All this helps me feel healthier and happier, and that goes a long way. Can you recognize which foods bring you down and which ones make you feel upbeat and energized?

DO: GET OUT OF THE HOUSE
Get outdoors and into the sunshine for at least fifteen minutes a day, preferably forty-five minutes, especially in the morning. I have my dog to thank for ritualizing a morning walk, and I'm grateful. The National Sleep Foundation explains that going outside regulates your

circadian rhythms, which impact sleep, mood, and energy levels. Sunlight also helps your body produce vitamin D, which is necessary for the absorption of calcium. Vitamin D deficiency has also been linked to depression, lowered immune function, heart disease, and diabetes. Your doctor can check your levels in a routine blood test during your annual physical. Being outside can also help combat the "winter blues." Six times as many women as men suffer from the more severe type of winter-related depression, seasonal affective disorder (SAD), according to the Mayo Clinic. One of my daughters developed SAD when she went to school in New Hampshire. The long winters (and sometimes eight feet of snow!) were brutal. We bought her a light therapy box for her desk and it really helped. Get some sun!

DON'T: STAY UP ALL NIGHT

When you're sleeping too little, your mood suffers. The average adult needs between seven and a half and eight hours of sleep a night. Some studies suggest that women need more sleep than men because our multitasking brains literally work harder and need more time to wind down at night. If you are having trouble sleeping, avoid alcohol and caffeine, keep your room dark and cool, and power down your electronic devices at least an hour before bedtime. Research shows that blue screens reduce the output of melatonin, the hormone that regulates sleep. Honesty check: I don't do this, but I know I should. My cell phone is inches from my bed, and I compulsively check it if I wake up in the middle of the night and certainly first thing in the morning. I'll try to stop doing this if you will. I do have a sleep routine, though;

it's boring but it works for me: herbal tea, comfortable pajama, and a book.

Or there's always this option:

> At seventy years old, if I could give my younger self one piece of advice, it would be to use the words 'fuck off' much more frequently.
>
> —HELEN MIRREN

DO: TRY MEDITATION EVEN IF IT SEEMS WEIRD AND IMPOSSIBLE

I used to tease my husband about his meditation practice (which he annoyingly—to me at least—refers to as "sitting"), but after six months I suddenly noticed that he was significantly less prone to anger and moodiness. He swears that it also sharpens his intellect and has helped him cope with some very stressful life events. There is mounting scientific research on the wonders of meditation, which include slowing the brain's aging process, quieting the mind to reduce stressful thoughts, combatting depression and anxiety, and improving concentration.

It can seem like an esoteric practice, and you might not know where to begin, but there are lots of resources to help you get started. You can use guided meditations. Again, Tara Brach (she has a user-friendly website and free podcasts) is wise, accessible, and funny. There are also a number of highly rated apps, including Headspace and the Mindfulness App. Though it only takes twenty minutes a day to start reaping the benefits, if you want to dive in, you could take a class (many yoga studios now offer them) or sign up for a retreat.

DON'T: SACRIFICE THINE SELF FOR EVERYBODY ELSE

When I took an informal poll among my girlfriends asking about what was essential for self-care, the number one response was time alone. We just don't get enough of it. Between work and kids and friends and partners, women, particularly women at midlife, are totally swamped and at the mercy of everyone else. It's imperative to find time for self-reflection, self-love, and just plain peace, whatever that means to you.

Recently my friend Jodie broke a dinner date with me. She explained that her boyfriend, Sam (both twice divorced, a late-in-life passion), was out of town, and it was so rare for her to be alone in her house that she was just desperate to soak up the solitude. I totally got it. I'm almost always happy (thrilled, even!) when people cancel on me—it means a window of unexpected free time during which I can read a book or meditate or stare out the window (or go on the Internet, watch a movie, talk on the phone with my kids). Whatever feels replenishing—the point is that we need to prioritize me time. Downtime. We need to make space to check in with ourselves, to nurture ourselves, to breathe alone.

DO: FIND PURPOSE

Sometimes all I need is a little diversion to help me feel like myself again. A night out with friends at a bar or a hop on my pink bicycle to run errands in the neighborhood. Actions like these may not erase the gloom, but they do give me a bit of perspective and remind me that there are activities and people out there that I love. But, down deep, distractions aren't enough.

Yes, I saved the hardest one for last: what really makes the ultimate difference in my well-being is feeling useful, feeling functional, feeling like I'm doing something that has greater meaning. "Find purpose" may strike the cynical among you as a cheesy cliché, but I promise you, it's so not. Discovering what makes you want to get up in the morning, well…that's what makes you get up in the morning. When I'm really down, I can't always see those things for the fog, and it can help to make a list. Why am I here? In what ways am I a good force in the world?

The list is always changing, but here's mine right now:

1. Being alive (unlike my mother at this stage) to help my college-age children navigate the path to adulthood. Every thrill, every fear, every demand for money, these are all things I experienced, but I had no one to turn to at their age, and I'm so grateful every day that I can be their guiding star, however much I annoy them.

2. I'm a leader among my friends, and I take pride in being an organizer and (hopefully, sometimes) an inspiration. I want to help women thrive in their later years, and it feels great to talk about our hopes and fears aloud, to make it funny and real and to not hide behind shame.

3. I'm grateful to have romantic love in my life, and I hope to do it well, or better, before I die. If a challenge is a purpose, that's mine.

4. I love creating beautiful spaces for my friends and family to live in. Good, comfortable design feeds me, and I believe it feeds others, even if they don't know it.

5. I mentor a teenage girl who loves to write, and I can see that I'm teaching her things. Helping her makes me feel like I can make a difference in a hard life, and that gives me a great sense of purpose.
6. I love my dog.

What are yours?

Nobody will protect you from your suffering. You can't cry it away or eat it away or starve it away or walk it away or punch it away or even therapy it away. It's just there, and you have to survive it. You have to endure it. You have to live through it and love it and move on and be better for it and run as far as you can in the direction of your best and happiest dreams across the bridge that was built by your own desire to heal.

—CHERYL STRAYED, *TINY BEAUTIFUL THINGS: ADVICE ON LOVE AND LIFE FROM DEAR SUGAR*

CHAPTER SEVEN

(HEALTH)

NOT WHAT THE DOCTOR ORDERED

The really frightening thing about middle age is the knowledge that you'll grow out of it.
—DORIS DAY

MY MOTHER WAS THIRTY-SEVEN and a single mother of two young kids when she was first diagnosed with breast cancer in 1980. She had a lumpectomy but opted out of chemotherapy and radiation in favor of homeopathic medicines, meditation, and adhering to a macrobiotic diet. Do you remember the eighties tome *The Cancer Prevention Diet* by Michio Kushi? That was my mother's bible. For breakfast she *drank* the liquid her vegetables had steamed in the night before! She also ran ten miles three times a week, for whatever good that did her. When her cancer recurred four years later, she made the same unconventional treatment choice, and I'll never know why, because it was never discussed. She opted to keep her cancer a secret throughout my childhood. When it returned for the third and last time when I was nineteen, the chemotherapy to which she finally acquiesced was not enough to save her.

I spent much of my twenties and thirties pathologically afraid I'd get breast cancer one day. I started having mammograms when I was twenty-seven (conventional wisdom then was to start ten years before your mother's age of onset), and now, twenty years later, I'm on a six-month checkup routine—a breast MRI in the fall and a mammogram every spring. I've had two benign (knock on wood) breast biopsies, one surgical and one needle, and I've taken the BRCA test twice (no mutation detected), ten years apart. I did it the second time because there was so much more research. In other words, I try to stay on top of it as much as I can. And as scared as I am every time I go for a screening, I remind myself that knowledge is power.

My breast cancer may be your Alzheimer's or diabetes or osteoporosis. By this time in our lives, we've all encountered disease and infirmity, and usually we each have particular afflictions we fear more than others based on our personal life experience and family history. There are some diseases we'll be more or less genetically predisposed to and others that perhaps we can ward off with lifestyle choices, but in the end, there's a lot we can't control. The reality is, the things we fear most may likely never happen. But no doubt, other stuff will! While anyone can get cancer at any age—according to the American Cancer Society, more than 1.5 million new cancer cases are diagnosed each year—the risk goes up with age, and nearly nine out of ten cancers are diagnosed in people ages fifty and older. This is just one small part of health and aging; we are also going to start having awful but non-life-threatening aches and pains and conditions, and it will suck.

For example, I never had vaginal dryness, and then one day at forty-six, I experienced pain during sex. I thought I had combatted it with major lubricant action (see chapter two), and then, a year later, at forty-seven, it came back, but this time in the form of bladder pain and a need to pee every two seconds. As I type, I have to pee, and I'm praying this goes away and doesn't become a chronic condition. I'm told I need topical estrogen, and that this is a very common ailment many women our age experience. It's not cancer, surely, but the prospect of feeling like I have a bladder infection for the rest of my life is pretty goddamn depressing. I can't read a menu or a shampoo bottle without glasses, and I'm starting to worry about my hearing. I have two male friends with prostate cancer, one with MS, lots of friends who can no longer run or hike because of injuries . . . all the usual complaints of age-related wear and tear on our bodies: the physical aspect of the human condition. So what's a woman to do?

Note: with all health-related issues and suggestions, research and recommendations are constantly being updated. Please refer to the "Notes and Resources" section for well-vetted websites with the most current information.

WHAT'S UP, DOC?

FINDING THE RIGHT DOCTOR IS A big issue that we don't talk or think about enough. Some of us have moved a lot, so we've switched doctors a million times. Some of us have crappy insurance and hate everyone on our plan. Some of us loved the guy or gal who delivered our babies, but now that person has retired (I loved looking up to my older doc as a mother figure when I was young, but now I'm old and she's dead!) and we find ourselves at fifty without a regular doctor. Very few of us, I'm sure, have felt taken care of by a consistent team or even one person who we feel truly knows our bodies and our cares and concerns and can guide us through menopause and into older age. This is a problem with the American health care system—I'm sure you've noticed that life isn't great for most doctors anymore either, scrambling from one patient to the next to make ends meet while dealing with the enormous hassles of electronic medical records and insurance companies. But never does it feel like a bigger problem than when you actually have something wrong with your body. It's terrifying to feel sick and unsure and not have a professional you trust. And yet, it happens all the time.

I don't have any great answers. I know it's complicated and getting even harder. But I do think even being aware that this is a problem can help. *Think* about who your doctors are and whether you trust them. Do they answer your questions thoroughly or brush you off? Do they call you back in a crisis? If not, start asking friends and do research. Really make an effort to find at least one medical professional you feel good about, and start to develop a relationship. I feel fortunate that I have the cell phone numbers of both my internist and my gynecologist, and in a crisis I don't think twice about texting them. The level of comfort you can get from a medical professional who cares is huge, and comfort equals a measure of stress relief, which we all know is high on the list of what makes us feel sane.

CAN ANYONE PLEASE EXPLAIN HRT TO ME?!

IT'S HARD TO OVERSTATE HOW MUCH declining estrogen messes with our bodies, and lately I feel like every day brings a new treat. Like me, you're very likely to notice some symptoms—whether it's hot flashes, insomnia, bone loss, weight gain, anxiety, bladder pressure, and so on—in your late forties, and certainly by your fifties. The question here is WTF can we do about it? What's safe, what's advisable, what's necessary? Particularly when it feels like your body is a moving target, hormone levels are changing incessantly, and frankly, I don't have the time or money to be getting my blood tested every other week.

If you ask ten women over fifty—and even more confusing, if you ask ten different doctors—you're equally likely to get ten different answers. The only thing everyone seems to agree on is that losing estrogen screws with your body and the only real solution aside from grinning and bearing it is hormone replacement therapy. You'll hear suggestions about treatments as varied as the ring, the patch, the cream, the gel, the birth control pill, antidepressants, exercise, and grin and bear it. Some rave about bioidenticals, and others still seem to be using your grandmother's Premarin, which comes from horse's urine. It can be dispiriting to realize that there is simply no one answer. You really do have to sift through the information and make your own best evaluation, or choose the doctor who you think seems the smartest and follow his or her advice. I'm not a doctor and am not dispensing medical advice, but here's a bit of history, and a summary of what I know and have done, as well as what my trusted girlfriends are saying.

Premarin, a synthetic estrogen made from the urine of pregnant mares, was first marketed in 1942, the year my mother was born. For decades this was the standard treatment to help keep women looking and feeling young (skin youthful, bones strong, heart disease at bay), but over time research showed an increase in uterine cancer for women who were using this therapy, and then Prempro, a synthetic progestin, was added to the standard mix. Doctors were trained that HRT was a no-brainer for women over fifty.

Then, in 2002, a research study from the Women's Health Initiative found that taking HRT (estrogen plus progestin) significantly increased a woman's risk of heart disease and breast cancer. I remember being a young breastfeeding mom when the study was published and seeing it splashed all over the front of the *New York Times*. A second WHI study published two years later reinforced the message, finding that taking estrogen alone also increased the risk of stroke, dementia, and other serious health problems. Almost overnight the number of women using HRT dropped by nearly half. So, I grew into middle age inferring from the zeitgeist that all hormone treatments were evil and toxic and just assumed I would eschew them. It was surprising and confusing to then hit perimenopause and start to learn that my friends were all over the map on this issue and that plenty of them were using, are using, or are starting to use *some* form of hormone treatment, out of either vanity (moist skin, please!) or real desperation (hot flashes that make going to work almost impossible) or pressing health concerns (my bladder issue, for example).

Premarin is a natural hormone—if your native food is hay!

—DR. JOEL HARGROVE

Luckily for all of us, there do seem to be some safe options now, within parameters. Today, many years and many studies after the 2002 news, our good friends at the North American Menopause Society (NAMS) tell us that we need not worry so much. It may *seem* like no one agrees on the subject of hormone therapy, but they insist that the experts do agree on the key points.

NAMS, the American Society for Reproductive Medicine, and the Endocrine Society all currently take the position that healthy, recently menopausal women can use hormone therapy for relief of their symptoms of hot flashes and vaginal dryness if they so choose.

- HRT is most effective for symptoms like hot flashes and vaginal dryness. If you have only vaginal dryness, the preferred treatment is low doses of vaginal estrogen. But why not try coconut oil or lube first!

- Women who still have a uterus need to take a progestogen (progesterone or a similar product) along with the estrogen to prevent uterine cancer. Five years or less is generally the recommended duration of use for this combined treatment.

- Women who have had their uterus removed can take estrogen alone, and because of the apparent greater safety of estrogen alone, there may be more flexibility in how long women can safely use estrogen therapy.

- Both estrogen therapy and estrogen with progestogen therapy increase the risk of blood clots in the legs and lungs, similar to birth control pills, patches, and rings. Although the risks of blood clots and strokes increase with either type of hormone therapy, the risk is rare in the fifty to fifty-nine age group.

- An increased risk in breast cancer is seen with five or more years of continuous estrogen/progestogen therapy, possibly earlier. The risk decreases after hormone therapy is stopped. Use of estrogen alone for an average of seven years in the Women's Health Initiative trial did not increase the risk of breast cancer.

- There is a lack of safety data supporting the use of hormone therapy in women who have had breast cancer. Nonhormonal therapies should be the first approach in managing menopausal symptoms in breast cancer survivors.

This essentially echoes what my doctor has told me, which is that HRT is safe if done early (up to age fifty-nine or within ten years of menopause) and for not too long (five years), for women who are otherwise healthy and have not had cancer. Individualization is key to this decision; you have to weigh quality-of-life priorities as well as personal risk factors such as age, time since menopause, and risk of blood clots, heart disease, stroke, and breast cancer. With my family history of breast cancer, the idea of taking hormones scares me to no end. On the other hand, how long do I want to live with painful sex, hot flashes, and thinning hair?

AND WHAT ARE THESE THINGS CALLED BIOIDENTICAL HORMONES?

BIOIDENTICAL HORMONES, often touted as a superior form of HRT, are hormones that are made from a plant chemical extracted from yams and soy, and they are the exact chemical replica of what is produced in the body. Compare this to Premarin, for example, which comes from a "natural" source, mares' urine, but has a different chemistry, containing a dozen estrogen compounds, only one of which is a replica of what we produce in the human body, while the others are foreign to us. Soybeans and yams contain unique compounds that can exactly replicate what we make in our bodies, but, sadly, we can't get this benefit from just eating them.

There is a lot of confusion around the definitions of "natural" versus that of "bioidentical" versus that of "synthetic," and the basic thing to remember is that "bioidentical" refers to the shape of the molecule itself rather than the source of the hormone. Anything can be (and often is) legally marketed as "natural" or "plant based" but still not be anywhere near "bioidentical" to human female hormones.

I didn't even take chemistry in high school, let alone study medicine, so I'm not advocating for anything here, just trying to give you a sense of the terrain in layman's terms. What I can say about bioidenticals is that women's health guru Christiane Northrup, MD, recommends them. A Beverly Hills doctor by the name of Uzzi Reiss offers a compelling argument in his book *Natural Hormone Balance for Women.* My own doctor, Laura Corio, author of the so-well-titled *The Change Before the Change,* is a huge proponent, and if that isn't enough for you, in her incarnation as a menopause maven, Suzanne Somers swears by them. If it's good enough for Chrissy, it's good enough for me.

PERIMENOPAUSE LASTS HOW LONG?

A study says owning a dog makes you ten years younger.
My first thought was to rescue two more, but I don't want to go through menopause again.
—JOAN RIVERS

DANA: I've reached the stage of perimenopause where I am totally unpredictable except that I am still getting a period—it can be thirty-eight days or twenty-two. I feel twelve years old again, like I have to walk around and check my panties every time I pee (and I can no longer, at forty-seven, rely on things like my lower back aching to clue me in, as it seems to ache all the time these days—sigh!). SO READY for this shit to be OVER! Just how long does this fun stage usually last?

Sadly, Dana, the average length of perimenopause is four years, but apparently it can last up to ten years! Almost as long as prepubescent childhood! It generally starts with irregular periods; then the crazy myriad symptoms pile on in spurts and starts and often with unexpected twists and turns, until finally you'll notice that you haven't had a period for a full twelve months. At that point you can consider yourself off the train. But that doesn't mean that symptoms like hot flashes will disappear. In fact, according to my friend Sarah's gynecologist, "They may get worse." Sorry.

DEAR LORD, PLEASE DON'T TRY TO SELL ME ANOTHER SUPPLEMENT

WHEN I FIRST STARTED HAVING HOT flashes and waking up at four a.m., I went out and bought one of those handy pill dispensers with a box for each day of the week. Feeling very efficient, I then skipped off to my local health food store, convinced somehow that buying a sack of vitamins and supplements would be life changing. I spent hundreds of dollars on black cohosh, evening primrose, dong quai, flaxseed, red clover, wild yam, ginseng, St. John's wort, and DHEA.

Two months later I found myself on the examination table with my internist, crying about how tired I was. She gently told me that the things I was taking were totally useless and offered me an antidepressant and the birth control pill. I didn't take her up on either because I decided to do more research, but her take on supplements was confirmed for me by a paper written by JoAnn Pinkerton, executive director of NAMS. It's tellingly titled "Don't DIY with Herbs and Supplements for Menopause," and Pinkerton states very clearly that aside from *maybe* soy foods and supplements (and only for those women whose bodies can use soy to produce a compound called equol), no other herb or supplement shows an effect any greater than a placebo. Not only are they not helpful, but some may be dangerous. Black cohosh, for example, may cause liver damage, and a lot of the yam creams out there have been adulterated with steroids and synthetic estrogen- and progesterone-type compounds. The University of Maryland Medical Center backs that up and says that, at best, yam creams have a mild placebo effect.

Don't waste your money!

LEAKY LADY PARTS: INCONTINENCE AND OTHER URINARY DISASTERS

I'VE TALKED A LOT ABOUT the benefits of exercise, and it is wonderful, until you notice the big pee stain blooming in the crotch of your leggings. A woman whom I jog with told me how fed up she was with her ongoing incontinence issues. "It started after I had my first baby. When he was about four months old, I was psyched to go out for my first run. A few minutes in, my nylon jogging shorts were soaked. Nobody had warned me about this. I felt so discouraged!" And she's been dealing with it for the last nineteen years. According to a study from UC Davis that analyzed nine years of data from three thousand women ages forty-two to sixty-four, nearly 70 percent of us pee on ourselves at least once a month. Ugh.

There are a plethora of issues leading to incontinence:

1. Good ol' urinary incontinence. Incontinence, or what's referred to as an "overactive bladder," can develop as a result of pelvic floor muscles and nerves being stretched or damaged during childbirth and just plain aging. The two kinds are called stress incontinence, where you pee upon sneezing or coughing or exercising, and urge incontinence, when the muscles around the bladder put pressure on the organ at inconvenient times or with too much urgency. According to Harvard Medical School guidelines, you can take medication for incontinence and even get surgery, but the latest recommendations from the American College of Physicians are lifestyle-related treatments, which they claim have about a 70 percent rate of effectiveness. Strength training the muscles of the pelvic floor improves stress incontinence. Bladder training (learning to use the bathroom on a schedule) is effective for urgency issues. Losing weight can help women who are classified as overweight or obese (extra pounds put pressure on the lower abdominal muscles and organs). You can also try to minimize "bladder irritants," which are all things we enjoy, like alcohol, spicy foods, caffeine, and citrus fruits.

2. Apparently thinning vaginal walls due to estrogen depletion can cause an overactive bladder, which involves a literal nonstop urge to pee (as in, minutes after flushing, you're headed back to the john), particularly worse at night for some reason. (This even has a medical term, nocturia!) This happened to me and it

was a nightmare. I thought I had a UTI—it seemed obvious with the pain and urgency, so I requested antibiotics over the phone from my doc, who complied. It was only ten days later, when I was still suffering from symptoms, and mostly at night only, that I started to worry it was something else. I called her back and described what was going on, and also got a urine culture, which confirmed no infection—and she diagnosed an estrogen issue and prescribed Estrace. Within days I felt human again.

3. But it could also be a urinary tract infection. Remember when you just got these because you had so much hot, dirty sex? Well now you may get them because older women simply do… with more frequency than the rest of the population. Thinner tissues, which may be irritated tissues after sex, contribute to the problem, which is an excellent reason for lots more foreplay (and lube up!). If you do think you have a UTI, make sure you get a culture, and don't just self-diagnose, like I did.

4. Pelvic floor dysfunction. Did you know that there's a whole field of physical therapy devoted to strengthening the pelvic floor? In women, the pelvic floor consists of the muscles, ligaments, connective tissues, and nerves that support the bladder, uterus, vagina, and rectum and help these pelvic organs work properly. Generally thought to be caused by childbirth, pelvic floor dysfunction covers a wide range of issues that can occur when the "sling," or "hammock," that supports the pelvic organs becomes weak or damaged. The three main types of pelvic floor disorders are: lack of bladder control, lack of bowel control, and pelvic organ prolapse, a condition in which the uterus, bladder,

or bowel may "drop" and push into the vaginal canal. According to one study I read, funded by the National Institutes of Health, almost one-quarter of women face pelvic floor disorders—that's 27 percent of women ages forty to fifty-nine, 37 percent of women ages sixty to seventy-nine, and nearly half of women age eighty or older! That's a helluva lot of us for something no one talks about, don't you think?

5. Interstitial cystitis, aka painful bladder syndrome, is one of my biggest fears now that I've had a taste of this issue: a chronic condition causing bladder pressure, bladder pain, and sometimes pelvic pain. The pain ranges from mild discomfort to severe. The way it's been explained to me is that our bladders are like hot-water bottles. They expand until they are full and then signal your brain that it's time to pee, communicating through the pelvic nerves. With interstitial cystitis, which most often affects women, these signals get mixed up—you feel the need to pee more often and with smaller volumes of urine than considered normal. There's no cure, and you can imagine this can have some pretty awful ramifications on your quality of life, but I have been told that diet and physical therapy can offer relief.

Bottom line? These problems are crazy common and *never* talked about! If you are nodding in recognition or horror, or both, here are some voices from the trenches, so you know you are not alone:

> ***HILLARY:*** I need to discuss incontinence. After having three children, it was not uncommon to pee just a

little when I laughed really hard or sneezed or coughed super-loud. But I've noticed lately that there's an urgency to going to the bathroom that I've never experienced before. The other night I was riding my bike home after a dinner out, and it occurred to me about half the way to my house that I really had to go to the bathroom. By the time I got home it was bordering on disastrous. One minute more, and I would have peed all over myself. It really freaked me out. There are certainly many times during the course of any given week when you can't get to the bathroom when you need to, and I'm terrified of being in the position where that actually matters. Is anyone else experiencing this? Does anyone know what to do about this? HELP!!!

FELICIA: Actually, this was such an acute problem that my doctor sent me to a gyno-urologist, who then referred me to a vaginal physical therapist. I didn't go— mainly because of time—but I may need to revisit.

HILARY: Since having children, I've absolutely had slight incontinence on a jump, sneeze, etc. and there have definitely been times I had to go and held it in 'til painful.

LAURALEE: Try reducing your caffeine intake—it's a bladder irritant.

MARGARET: It is possible you have a condition known as interstitial cystitis. I suffered for years, thinking I was having bladder infections, constantly going on antibiotics, only to find out it was not an infection but rather a condition of the lining of the bladder. And yes, thinning of the tissues exacerbates the condition. I found relief with a combo of a change in diet and topical estrogen.

LAURA: What worked for the bladder for me was nettle tea and a tablespoon of raw unfiltered apple cider vinegar a few times a day until the Macrobid kicked in. It's just super-important to pee before and after sex and use coconut oil as an antibacterial.

LISA: I put coconut oil in my va-jj every night to help re the thinning walls. It's helped. And a sexologist I know says to put a small vibrator in there daily for 10 minutes, which stimulates blood flow to the area, also helps with the thinning walls.

If you have one of the above issues, I'm sorry. The solution may be as simple as antibiotics and cranberry juice, or nettle tea, or topical estrogen, or pelvic floor exercises. If your problem is beyond the ken of your gynecologist, you may need to consult a urogynecologist or a pelvic floor physiotherapist, both specialists in this field. They can fully assess your pelvic floor function and teach you appropriate techniques to strengthen it and train the bladder.

THE BIG SQUEEZE

WE'VE ALL HEARD A MILLION TIMES that Kegels are important for pelvic floor health (if vaginal prolapse isn't a scary concept, I don't know what is, even to a twentysomething), for sexual health (um, yeah), and for general core fitness, but how many of us actually ever do them? And if we do, are we doing them right?

What you don't want to do is exercise your pelvic floor by constantly stopping your pee. This is what a girlfriend's ninety-five-year-old grandfather, who enrolled in medical school before women got the vote, once recommended after she had her first baby. You may have heard the same advice from a more current source as well, but the American Pregnancy Association warns, "Don't do this too often during urination because it can actually weaken the muscles over time and/or increase your chance of a urinary infection." They suggest that you try it a couple of times only to get a sense of where your pelvic floor muscles even are.

Last year I spent $200 on a pale green gadget called the Elvie, which you connect via Bluetooth to your smartphone and stick up your vag and squeeze. This is one way to work on these muscles, but after using it twice (it's not nearly as fun as a vibrator but has the same element of secrecy and slight embarrassment), the novelty wore off. I moved on to an app called Kegel Camp, which I adore. Twice a day, at two p.m. and five p.m., an alarm goes off on my phone reminding me to Kegel. I never actually do it, or maybe just once when the alarm goes off, but still, it's a great idea. For the more diligent among us, when the alarm goes off you can open the app and spend five or ten minutes following the cheerful instructions. Other suggestions for making Kegels a regular habit? One of my girlfriends does them every time she's in an elevator. I also find that just texting the word "Kegel" to a friend every now and then is a great little way of saying I love you.

BEYOND THE KEGEL

Woolfer Lauren Ohayon, a yoga teacher, pelvic floor dysfunction expert, and the founder of the Restore Your Core strengthening program, provided me with this basic self-assessment for anyone experiencing incontinence, painful sex, or other related issues.

Optimize Your Pelvic Floor Checklist

If you leak pee, have painful sex, sneeze pee, or have any other pelvic floor issue that you are chalking up to age, it is likely not an age issue and, yes, it can get better. Ohayon warns that a myriad of factors, from breathing mechanics to high heels ("death" to the pelvic floor) to even doing too many Kegels, can contribute to less than optimal conditions in your pelvic floor muscles. The good news is that we are not stuck with these issues. Here is what she advises you do for optimal function:

1. **Work on having a well-balanced and functional body:** When our muscular system is compromised, our pelvic floor takes a

big hit. Crucial to the health of the pelvic floor is having a good balance of the muscles that affect it, namely your leg and hip musculature. The program includes mindfully executed squats, lunges, and other lower-body exercises.

2. **Alignment:** When we are out of alignment, our muscles become compromised. A big factor in pelvic floor issues is when our hips habitually shift forward and the side hip is no longer stacked over the knee and the ankle. This is very common! You will know this is happening because when you stand you have a lot of weight in the front of your foot as opposed to your heels. When our hips shift forward, our pelvic floor muscles tighten to support us there. Look at your alignment in a mirror (in profile). If you dangle a yoga strap or belt from your hip to your foot, it will show you if your hips are stacked properly over your ankle and your legs are perpendicular to the floor or if your pelvis is thrust forward, creating a diagonal from hip to ankle joint.

3. **Breathing:** Believe it or not, chronic belly breathing puts a ton of pressure on our pelvic floor. Learning to breathe more into the ribs will greatly reduce pressure on the pelvic floor.

4. **Sit less, change position more, move around more:** Sitting a lot makes the muscles of our legs, pelvic floor, and core adapt to being used in shortened positions, which in turn compromises the pelvic floor.

5. **Corrective exercises:** There are a bunch of fantastic corrective exercises that can help rebalance the muscles of the pelvic floor. Seeking out a physical therapist or a personal trainer to help you assess your muscular imbalances and give you a set of corrective exercises and breath work is essential to resolving pelvic floor issues.

And BTW, my friend Samantha followed Ohayon's tips for eight weeks and no longer pees while jogging!

Lifestyle changes and exercise won't work immediately, so in the meantime, you need to find the best, comfiest protection. Studies have shown that the majority of women with incontinence use sanitary napkins to help them get through the day, but period protection is actually inadequate. It turns out that the science of menstrual flow absorption is different from that of urine absorption! The permeable top layer of a pad typically pulls blood moisture into the underlying absorbent layer, away from your skin, and while this effectively keeps your skin dry, it's not made to handle the chemical composition of urine. Urine soaking a sanitary napkin can actually be damaging to the skin, and specifically designed incontinence pads and underwear are designed to absorb the rapid dispersion of pee. Some incontinence pads have special gels that not only draw urine away from the top layer, but also change it to a more solid substance. This neutralizes the potentially harmful chemical composition of pee. Others have polymer fabrics with wicking capabilities that also draw moisture from the top layer, eliminating urine odor and neutralizing pH levels to limit the risk of skin breakdown. Who knew?! Luckily for us, Depends is no longer the only option.

Always brand makes some products for this issue, and for the super-stylish among us, there is now a whole line of glamorous incontinence underwear called Icon. You may have seen the ads on social media: sleek pee-proof bikinis and boy shorts worn by fit gray-haired models doing complicated yoga poses. They are expensive (around $30 a pair) but if you add it up, so are pads. My jogging buddy, who had been using minipads almost daily for years, rotates two pairs for working out. She had used panty liners, which barely did the trick but at least weren't bulky or chafing like thicker pads. She says her Icon panties work better, have flat seams so they are pretty much invisible even under leggings, and are more comfortable. She just rinses them out in the shower after a run and hangs to dry.

Lastly, don't be afraid to talk about incontinence. Women often don't bring it up with their doctors because they are embarrassed, and they don't know that it can be treated when in fact it's really, really common, and there are so many solutions. Talk about it, look around, ask your friends. Don't suffer in quiet shame.

WILL I EVER SLEEP THROUGH THE NIGHT AGAIN?

HONESTLY? IT'S NOT LOOKING GOOD. A survey done in 1995 by the National Institute on Aging looked at nine thousand men and women aged sixty-five and older and found that 42 percent of them reported difficulty with both falling asleep and staying asleep.

A chapter in Annabelle Gurwitch's hilarious book *I See You Made an Effort* gives us a sample of what's going through all of our menopausal minds when we're awake at four a.m., and it had me on the floor laughing.

FROM ANNABELLE GURWITCH'S HILARIOUS BOOK, *I SEE YOU MADE AN EFFORT*:

The Four A.M. Club

JILL: It's not enough. I'm not a good enough parent. Holocaust. I'm so sick of myself. I hope I can fall back to sleep.

GIA: If I could just lose those ten pounds... would more people come to my funeral?

MAUREEN: I hate this pillow... I also hate this pillow... Why don't I have any good pillows? I will probably never be able to afford to go to Venice before it sinks into the water or I'll be too old to enjoy it. As I lie here not sleeping, I'm getting fatter. Why didn't I take some kind of computer programming class? Please let me live til my kid becomes a grown-up. My joints hurt—is that arthritis? Or cancer? Or menopause? Or because I spent hours walking up and down the aisles at Costco buying things I didn't need? What's the least amount of money I need to live on?

MAGGIE: If I watch some porn, will my kids wake up and walk in on me?

SUSAN: I dream that I am looking in the mirror and notice a couple long chin hairs. As I look closer, it becomes dozens of really long hairs, so much so that I look like Fu Manchu. I am distressed thinking that I've been walking around like this for who knows how long and no one bothered to tell me. Then I come up with the idea that to spare the expense of having to get my face waxed, maybe I could just wrap it around my neck like a scarf. I wake up convinced it wasn't a dream, but reality. I have to check the mirror several times to make sure I'm not wearing a head scarf.

CAROL: This would be the perfect time to go through my husband's phone and email.

For women, the problem typically starts in early perimenopause, and then unfortunately it increasingly gets worse as we transition into later menopause. In a 2016 study from the University of Pennsylvania, researchers found that 31 to 42 percent of perimenopausal women reported symptoms that met the criteria for nighttime insomnia disorder, and that the numbers are worse for women whose menopause has been brought on by surgery.

Despite my skepticism about supplements, this is an area where some may actually help, and I report that from both personal and anecdotal experience.

MELATONIN, VALERIAN, AND THE MILLION OTHER THINGS PEOPLE TELL YOU TO TAKE

■ Try magnesium supplements and tart cherry juice, which is a natural source of melatonin. Or take the lowest dose of OTC melatonin. (One tablet contains many times what our bodies produce naturally.)

■ Pop the occasional Benadryl. It's been used safely for decades. And guess what? It contains the same active ingredient (diphenhydramine) found in Tylenol PM and many other OTC sleep aids without the addition of other ingredients such as acetaminophen, which are not great for your liver.

■ Discuss a sleeping pill Rx such as Ambien or Lunesta for short-term relief with your doctor. Or ask about an off-label prescription such as gabapentin, which is non-habit-forming and has been shown to reduce anxiety and may help with hot flashes. Another off-label option is the antidepressant trazadone. One girlfriend says simply having half a Klonopin on her bedside table "just in case" helps her sleep through the night (usually without taking it).

■ Try good old HRT—many friends say the estrogen patch makes all the difference.

■ Drink valerian tea before bed or try a tincture of skullcap (make sure it's the species *Scutellaria lateriflora*), which one friend swears by. Even herbal remedies can have dangerous interactions with alcohol or medications, so please do your research.

However, Dr. Jenny Breznay told me that while the tools in this list will be helpful for acute reactive insomnia (brought on by grief, for example, or serious stress), "for chronic insomnia, medications really don't work. What does work is CBT, cognitive behavioral therapy." She's referring to a complete retraining of your body and mode of thinking, which may mean things like not eating for a few hours before bed, keeping your room dark and free of technology, pushing yourself to not nap during the day, and making other changes.

Or you can get creative and chill out about the whole thing. Woolfer Marcia says, "Insomnia has been a part of my life since menopause. Only upside is fabulous conversations with other friends in the wee hours when no one can sleep!!! I have become accustomed to great beginnings and then 3 hours on/off. Learn a ton on public radio in those other wakeful moments. It's part of it all!!"

AND THEN THERE'S SNORING

MANY WOMEN I KNOW USE the word "kill" when it comes to talking about their husbands' snoring. Apparently, I'm in the minority here, because sleeping with my husband is probably my favorite thing about him. If either of us ever develops a snoring issue and feels the need to sleep in a separate room, that might literally be the death knell for the relationship. But for others, this is just another hurdle of growing old together. Recently, the Woolfers received an anonymous plea from a desperate woman:

> I need advice. Actually I need reassurance. I've had serious trouble sleeping ever since menopause. Not just insomnia some nights, but the inability to sleep when there's any noise, including snoring. Over the

past few months, my husband has gained a lot of weight. He's always been up and down, but now he's really up. And that increases his snoring so I'm really up—and stressed and anxious and angry—much of the night. So now I'm faced with two choices: sleep in the guest room, which makes him angry OR sleep without any real sleeping in our bedroom, which makes him happy but makes me miserable. I've chosen the guest room. But I feel so guilty and sad!

What I learned was that many couples are keeping each other up at night (not only men snore, of course), and quite a few are choosing to sleep separately. It's yet another dirty little secret that people don't talk about. We have this image that a solid, sexy relationship involves sleeping in each other's arms (maybe on red satin sheets, after perfect simultaneous orgasm). As my friend Sarah put it, "I feel like I'm outing myself with this. There's a lot of stigma. My husband snores and it ruins my sleep. We often sleep apart, especially on work nights, and when people discover this they act like our relationship must suck (it doesn't)." The general consensus was if one partner is torturing the other all night with snoring, moving to another bed or hitting the couch (or asking him or her to) is completely warranted. Men seem to be much more sensitive about this than women, and it can take high-level negotiating tactics to pull it off without hurt feelings. Maybe it's because they snore more and don't have to deal with the hell of waking up every hour and having to roll a crotchety person back onto his side as often as women do. Kate commented, "He might not understand just how hard it is for you to sleep. Ask him if you can tape a few minutes of what he sounds like to play back to him in the AM. I am sure he will be shocked, and if the situation was reversed, I doubt very much he could sleep."

Aside from sleeping apart, less drastic solutions include using a white noise machine or fan (I know one woman who lugs an industrial fan along when she and her husband travel!), buying good-quality earplugs, using a wedge pillow to keep him lying on his side, and trying over-the-counter nasal strips or a chin strap. However, snoring can also be a sign of a more serious health problem, and according to the Mayo Clinic, snoring that's loud enough to disrupt the sleep of your bedmate should be discussed with a doctor. If snoring is caused by obstructive sleep apnea (when your throat tissues partially block your airway) it can lead to irritability, grogginess, and even heart attack and stroke. It really is crucial to be evaluated by a specialist, who may recommend using a customized dental appliance or continuous positive airway pressure (CPAP) mask. The bottom line is that you don't have to put up with years of disturbed sleep: there is an answer!

THE CRUEL IRONY OF THE THREE P.M. SLUMP

ANDREA: Nodding off at desk. Daily.

ACCORDING TO THE National Sleep Foundation, more than 61 percent of women report having insomnia at some point in their lives, so I suspect that about the same number are also trashed by the time afternoon rolls around. You know that feeling, say an hour or two after lunch, when keeping your eyes open feels like work, and actual work feels downright impossible? When you find yourself wanting an espresso or a Snickers or a nap? A few things I've found that *might* help:

■ Eliminate sugar. Many studies have shown that intake of sugar decreases the activity of orexin cells, which are neuropeptides that regulate arousal and wakefulness.

■ Go gluten-free. A 2015 study, "Going Gluten-Free," from Aberdeen University's Rowett Institute of Nutrition and Health, the largest of this kind ever done in the UK, showed significant decrease in fatigue in participants who eliminated gluten.

■ Brew a cup of tea between eleven thirty and twelve; it's said to boost metabolism for the rest of the day.

■ Get your B_{12} and iron levels checked (although I did and mine were fine—still tired anyway).

■ Drink a huge glass of water (we're often not hydrated enough; this really can help).

■ Try a high-potency fish oil if you don't already eat oily fish regularly—omega-3s boost energy levels.

■ If you can swing it, *do* take a twenty-minute nap; besides just making you feel better, it actually reduces the risk of heart disease, amazingly enough. I read in *Variety* that Jill Soloway has a bed in her office on the Paramount lot! If she can nap, so can you.

WEATHER REPORT SAYS BRAIN FOG

COGNITIVE ISSUES LIKE BRAIN FOG ARE very common among women going through menopause, confirms Mary Rosser, MD, PhD, an ob-gyn at the Montefiore Women's Center in Scarsdale, New York. Speaking with *Everyday Health*, she explained, "This is something that is wide-ranging, but people are worried that they're developing dementia." Dr. Rosser added, "They rush to tell us their memory is declining, they can't concentrate, they're not as organized, and that they have a lower attention span."

I have to admit that of the dozens of perimenopausal woes I do suffer from, I can't say I've had brain fog. Yet. So far my mind (such as it is) still feels as sharp as it ever was, and I don't think I'm forgetting things, like many of the women I know are. My friend Robin loses her cell phone so often that she's taken to storing in her bra, and another friend admits to regularly mixing up her son's name with her dog's. Menopausal brain fog is a real thing. Women often fear they're going crazy or developing Alzheimer's, when in fact (at least I'm told), brain function usually returns to normal once menopause is over.

The good news is that in most cases, it's not early-stage dementia.

The symptoms are more often a normal part of menopause (hormones, hot flashes, insomnia!), or possibly a result of undiagnosed ADHD, Rosser says. There's also the fact that we have much more on our brains than we did when we were younger. According to the Harvard School of Public Health, our brains shed "unused" memories to make room for new ones to be stored, and men and women both appear more absentminded as they slide into middle age.

When it comes to lifestyle factors, taking care of yourself by exercising, eating healthily, getting enough sleep, and limiting alcohol and caffeine can help improve symptoms, according to Rosser. Drug options include antianxiety medications and antidepressants. There's also no shame in making lists, relying on your calendar alerts, or finding other tricks such as sending yourself emails to compensate for normal forgetfulness, no matter how much your children may mock you.

I DIDN'T SEE THAT ONE COMING: NEW HEALTH RISKS

IN MY TWENTIES AND THIRTIES I may have worried about my health a lot, but I didn't necessarily stick with the healthiest habits all the time—and it didn't seem to matter much. Scarfing my little kids' leftover mac and cheese or cupcakes, having the occasional cigarette, getting drunk, skipping workouts, staying up until two a.m.; my younger body bounced back in about two seconds. At our age, the necessity of vigilant health-buoying lifestyle behaviors hits you all of a sudden like a bowling ball, not only to look and feel good, but to actually avoid getting a chronic disease. When my friend Linda was forty-five she called me a little stunned after her annual physical. She had gained eight pounds, putting her in the "overweight" category, and her bad cholesterol was suddenly in the moderately high-risk range, as was her blood pressure. Her vitamin D and B$_{12}$ levels were also low and she said that she had been feeling exhausted and a little depressed for a few months. In the year since her last physical, when she had gotten a clean bill of health, she hadn't changed her eating or exercise routine in any dramatic way or faced exceptional stressors. She described how her doctor looked at her solemnly and asked her to think about where she would be in ten years if these numbers followed a steady trajectory.

There is no getting around the fact that the risk for certain diseases increases as a result of both hormonal changes (gee, thanks) and aging. While I'm not dispensing medical advice here, let's briefly run through some of the biggies.

THE BIG C

ACCORDING TO THE Centers for Disease Control, cancer is the number one killer of women over thirty-five. After sixty-five, cancer and heart disease alternate back and forth between numbers one and two in a morbid race to the finish. Breast, lung, and colorectal cancer are the three most common forms of the disease. Breast cancer is by far the most common, but lung cancer is the most deadly. To state the obvious: if you haven't quit smoking, this is the time to get serious about that. The CDC also encourages other lifestyle changes like limiting alcohol consumption, maintaining a healthy weight, managing other chronic diseases, and getting the recommended medical screenings.

HEALTH SCREENINGS CHEAT SHEET

SCREENING RECOMMENDATIONS ARE a moving target. One week the *New York Times* is telling you not to get a mammogram, and the next week an article will send you running to your doctor in fear. It's hard to keep up. Here are the current screening guidelines provided by the American Cancer Society:

BREAST CANCER

- Women ages 40 to 44 should have the choice to start annual breast cancer screening with mammograms if they wish to do so.

  "The choice"? Irritating.

- Women ages 45 to 54 should get mammograms every year.

- Women 55 and older should switch to mammograms every 2 years, or can continue yearly screening.

- Screening should continue as long as a woman is in good health and is expected to live 10 more years or longer.

I wonder how that expectation is assessed?

- All women should be familiar with the known benefits, limitations, and potential harms linked to breast cancer screening. They also should know how their breasts normally look and feel and report any breast changes to a health care provider right away.

Got it.

COLON AND RECTAL CANCER

Starting at age 50, both men and women should follow one of these testing plans:

- Colonoscopy every 10 years, or
- CT colonography (virtual colonoscopy) every 5 years, or
- Flexible sigmoidoscopy every 5 years, or
- Double-contrast barium enema every 5 years

In my case, I started at forty (because I had a friend who was diagnosed with stage-four rectal cancer and it scared me) and they found something bad—a flat precancerous polyp—when I was forty-five, so I'm really glad I did. Now I have to go every three years, so fun!

CERVICAL CANCER

■ Women between the ages of 30 and 65 should have a Pap test plus an HPV test (called "co-testing") done every 5 years.

■ Women over age 65 who have had regular cervical cancer testing in the past 10 years with normal results should not be tested for cervical cancer.

■ A woman who has had her uterus and cervix removed (a total hysterectomy) for reasons not related to cervical cancer and who has no history of cervical cancer or serious pre-cancer should not be tested.

ENDOMETRIAL/UTERINE CANCER

The American Cancer Society recommends that at the time of menopause, all women should be told about the risks and symptoms of endometrial cancer. Women should report any unexpected vaginal bleeding or spotting to their doctors.

LUNG CANCER

The American Cancer Society does not recommend tests to check for lung cancer in people who are at average risk. But, we do have screening guidelines for those who are at high risk of lung cancer due to cigarette smoking. Screening might be right for you if you are all of the following:

■ 55 to 74 years of age

■ In good health

■ Have at least a 30 pack-year smoking history AND are either still smoking or have quit within the last 15 years (A pack-year is the number of cigarette packs smoked each day multiplied by the number of years a person has smoked. Someone who smoked a pack of cigarettes per day for 30 years has a 30 pack-year smoking history, as does someone who smoked 2 packs a day for 15 years.)

Screening is done with an annual low-dose CT scan (LDCT) of the chest.

SKIN CANCER

Most skin cancers can be found early with skin exams. Exams by your doctor and checking your own skin frequently can help find cancers early, when they are easier to treat.

Regular skin exams are especially important for people who are at higher risk of skin cancer, such as people with reduced immunity, people who have had skin cancer before, and people with a strong family history of skin cancer.

It's important to check your own skin, preferably once a month (!), to look for new or abnormally shaped moles.

ADDITIONAL SCREENINGS

Depending on your health and family history and lifestyle behaviors, your doctor may suggest additional or more frequent tests for other potential issues, but more basics you don't want to forget are:

■ **Blood pressure.** High blood pressure is considered a "silent killer" because there are usually no symptoms. One of the last things you want to have is a stroke. Since it's free and easy, why not just get this tested every time you find yourself in a doctor's office?

■ **Cholesterol.** The American Heart Association recommends that all adults age twenty or older have their cholesterol and lipids checked every four to six years.

■ **Diabetes.** I'm sure you've heard that diabetes is a global epidemic, and at least three of my friends in their fifties have recently been told by their doctors that that they are "prediabetic," so this is really something to watch. The American Diabetes Association (ADA) recommends that adults age forty-five and older get screened for type 2 diabetes every three years.

■ Also, don't forget your **eyes and ears**! My vision feels like it's deteriorating by the day, and most eye-care experts recommend that you have a comprehensive eye exam every one to two years, depending on your age, risk factors, and whether you currently wear corrective lenses. I think I may have been ten the last time I had my hearing tested, but according to the Cleveland Hearing and Speech Center, by age sixty, everyone should have an initial, baseline evaluation. If hearing is found to be normal, then repeat evaluations every two to three years as recommended.

HEART DISEASE

WHILE MENOPAUSE DOES NOT CAUSE heart disease, the American Heart Association says that risk factors such as smoking and obesity begin to "take a toll" around this phase in women's lives. Once again, it's the loss of estrogen that is doing us in, although researchers are not sure of the exact correlation. The walls of our blood vessels become less flexible, making it easier for plaque and clots to form. There can also be an increase in the blood of a coagulant called fibrinogen. We need our blood to clot, but too much is dangerous and is considered an independent risk factor for coronary heart disease, myocardial infarction, and stroke—all of which we would really like to avoid!

An anonymous open letter to the group really drove home that it's imperative to take care of ourselves and scrutinize our priorities for the sake of our health:

An Open Letter to Mamas Who Do It All
(and What Mamas Don't?)

I'm forty-eight years old. I'm not overweight and I don't smoke or drink or have high blood pressure. If you don't count a tall, strong cup of coffee every morning and a small dark piece of chocolate most evenings, my diet is pretty reasonable. I am by no means an athlete or fitness buff, but I live a fairly active lifestyle and consider myself pretty healthy.

At least I did until last Tuesday, when I had a heart attack.

Sitting on my couch, gearing up for the dinner/homework/bedtime marathon, both of my kids otherwise engaged (that's momspeak for "having screen time"), I suddenly had a terrible case of heartburn. I recognized the pain, but this was worse and somehow different. I had read articles about how the classic grab-your-chest-left-arm-pain you imagine when you think "heart attack" isn't always the same for women. Yet I ignored the fact that I was experiencing chest pain and made sure everyone was taken care of before giving in to the pain and lying down to rest. Because that's what we, as mothers, tend to do, right? We push through. I mean, after pushing tiny humans out of your vagina, almost no pain is unbearable.

I sucked it up for more than twelve hours, and the next day, after getting my youngest off to school, I drove myself to the hospital.

Just moments after the words "heart" and "attack" were spoken, the doctor sat by my bedside and asked me, with a straight face, if I had been under any extreme stress lately. I took a short break from trying to figure out the logistics of who was going to pick up my son from school and get him to his after-school activity and shot the nice man a confused expression.

Really?

I have two children. And a job and a husband and an ex-husband and a mortgage and aging parents and in-laws and last week my older son totaled our only working car (he was fine), and oh yeah, a personal life. Who among us isn't under extreme stress? Add in any illness or other out-of-the-ordinary occurrence and it all falls apart.

Your load is probably different than mine, and I'm sure we all carry it in our own way, but damn if we don't all carry it. Ask any mother what happens when it all gets too heavy (and it always does) and something's got to give. The answer is always: us. We're the ones who give.

Motherhood is a precarious balancing act. A state of being constantly underwater. We paddle continuously and with very little regard for how tired it makes us. Our kids are sick? We work from home while holding the bucket. No food in the fridge? On it. Business is slow this month? I'll up my bookings. All while shouldering the burden of everyone else's issues. Even if we do find time for ourselves, it's not always enough to relieve the pressure.

I'm not here to tell you that you're doing it wrong, Dear Mamas. Absolutely, the kids need dinner and the work needs doing, the bills need paying and that laundry sure as hell isn't going to fold itself. Go ahead and do it all, but hear me when I tell you that you have to find a relief valve for yourself because it turns out that keeping everything together might be exactly the thing that undoes it all.

HIGH CHOLESTEROL

YOU KNOW HOW THEY ALWAYS TELL us that "good cholesterol"—high-density lipoprotein (HDL)—protects us women against atherosclerosis (the hardening of the arteries, which can lead to heart attacks and strokes)? Well, not so fast. According to a 2015 study from the University of Pittsburgh Graduate School of Public Health, these benefits are diminished during menopause as a result of hormonal alterations—especially estradiol reduction. "What we found is that, as women transition through menopause, increases in good cholesterol were actually associated with greater plaque buildup," Dr. Samar El Khoudary, assistant professor in Pitt Public Health's Department of Epidemiology, who served as the lead author for the study, reported at a meeting of the North American Menopause Society. "These findings suggest that the quality of HDL may be altered...thus rendering it ineffective in delivering the expected cardiac benefits." Even more confusing is that for some women, "bad cholesterol"—low-density lipoprotein (LDL)—may increase and

HDL may decrease, also a risk factor for atherosclerosis. Either way, this is not great news for us, and I'm not sure what else to say here, except to get your blood tested regularly and stay away from the foie gras!

CONDOMS: NOT JUST FOR TEENS

WOULDN'T YOU THINK THAT THE SILVER lining of your eggs drying up and your estrogen tanking would be never to have to look at a condom again? Alas, we still need to be mindful of STDs and getting pregnant. Most women have comforted at least one friend who is dealing with the misery of fertility treatment, but the flip side is that experts estimate that for women over forty, about half of pregnancies are unplanned. Of course the numbers are much lower, but don't assume that because you've missed a few periods and have fevered night sweats you can go bareback.

Brace yourself: more women in their forties and fifties are infected with the most common STD, trichomoniasis, than women in their twenties and thirties, according to a study by Johns Hopkins. Rates of other diseases such as syphilis, gonorrhea, chlamydia, and herpes are on the rise as well. The risk of contracting an STD can be exacerbated by thinning vaginal tissues and less natural lubrication. If you are divorced, dating, or otherwise on the market, I truly hope you are having the best, wildest, most uninhibited sex of your life, but unless you are certain you are in a monogamous relationship and your partner is STD-free, please heed the same advice you would give any young woman going off to college.

RHEUMATOID ARTHRITIS

MY KNEES HAVE BEEN CREAKY EVER since my period got erratic, and apparently this is not uncommon. Estrogen keeps inflammation down, and as it starts to drop off, joint pain is often a result (find more about this in chapter three). According to ob-gyn Marcelle Pick, the beginning of perimenopause is the first time many women complain about joint pain. You should eat oily fish, as omega-3s are thought to help with inflammation, but basically there's not a whole lot you can do about this. I'm letting you know it's normal. It *may* subside when your hormones settle down.

THYROID PROBLEMS

HOT FLASHES, INSOMNIA, MOOD CHANGES, low libido, hair loss: are your symptoms related to perimenopause or thyroid? Only a TSH test will tell. Your thyroid is a small bow-tie-shaped organ, located in the front of the neck above your collarbone. It produces hormones that regulate metabolism and frequently becomes dysfunctional (one in eight women between the ages of thirty-five and sixty-five have thyroid issues) in one of two ways:

■ Hypothyroidism (underactive thyroid) occurs when the thyroid no longer produces enough of the necessary hormones to keep the body functioning properly. If untreated, this can lead to high cholesterol, osteoporosis, heart disease, and depression.

■ Hyperthyroidism (overactive thyroid) occurs when the thyroid produces too much hormone. The most common signs are unusual weight loss, goiter (an enlarged thyroid gland), and exophthalmos (bulging eyes). Other symptoms can also mimic those of the menopause transition, including hot flashes, heat intolerance, palpitations (short episodes of rapid heartbeat), tachycardia (persistent rapid heartbeat), and insomnia.

Both conditions are very treatable and quite common, but you have to know to get tested. Also, be aware that not all endocrinologists agree on what levels are normal or abnormal, which can leave women with some confusion about how and when to treat.

Tips from our friends:

> *NANCY:* SUPER-IMPORTANT: the range of "normal" is wide! If you have symptoms, but are in the normal range, you might want to try meds for a month to see if you feel better. My "normal" is about a 1. My doctors

kept me at a 2 for years and I regret that—too tired to do much of anything fun for YEARS!

KATE: Yes, even within normal ranges you may be helped by getting further tests done if you have symptoms—many people are helped by taking good-quality vitamins since often women are low on D and B$_{12}$!

BONE HEALTH

WOOLFER LAURA NOTED A CONDITION that I had never heard of before. "My estrogen is really low. I'm going to an endocrinologist tomorrow because I just got my bone-density scan results back and on top of everything else I have osteopenia too! God it sucks to get old."

- Osteopenia refers to bone density that is lower than normal but not low enough to be classified as osteoporosis.

- Osteoporosis is the real deal—when the bones become brittle and fragile from loss of tissue, typically as a result of hormonal changes or deficiency of calcium or vitamin D. Many women with osteoporosis are prescribed bisphosphonates (brand names include Fosamax, Boniva, and Actonel) to prevent and treat bone loss.

You'll need a prescription to get a bone-density scan. While the U.S. Preventive Services Task Force recommends all women over sixty-five get one, my doc, Laura Corio, likes to get a baseline early and suggested I go soon, in my late forties.

GUM DISEASE AND OTHER FUNKY MOUTH PROBLEMS

I'M A LITTLE OCD ABOUT MY TEETH. I get them cleaned every three months now because every so often since my midforties, I spit out blood when I brush my teeth!

Yep. Turns out that the waxing and waning of good ol' estrogen during many phases of our female lives—starting with puberty, right through to pregnancy and then menopause—can affect how our gums react to plaque. Plaque and tartar buildup can cause the gums to swell and bleed. This is called gingivitis and can usually be combatted with good oral hygiene. When ignored, however, it can cause periodontal (gum) disease. Untreated periodontal disease can lead to all sorts of unspeakably horrible things like bone and tooth loss and even stroke, heart attack, and possibly even Alzheimer's disease.

The symptoms of periodontal disease include chronic bad breath, painful chewing, and red, swollen, tender, or bleeding gums that may pull away from the teeth. Apparently it's possible to have gum disease and not know it. My dentist, Marty Gottlieb, says, "Periodontal disease is a silent disease, but it's the number one cause of tooth loss. It doesn't always cause pain and discomfort. If you brush and your gums bleed, that's a sign of unhealthy gums. It also can cause the bone around the tooth to recede and you form a pocket where the toothbrush can't get in."

You know the drill: brush and floss regularly and schedule regular cleanings and checkups. Rinse your mouth with a baking soda solution to remove acid. Chew gum with xylitol (a sugar substitute made from sugar alcohol), which can decrease the bacteria that causes periodontal disease. If you are experiencing any of the symptoms described above, see your dentist, who might refer you to a periodontist.

Also, get this: in middle age, you might start noticing spots or lesions (totally benign, though) on the tongue, a condition called geographic tongue! Or you may feel a scalding sensation in your mouth, known as burning-mouth syndrome. Both are more common in women than in men.

DOES MY HUSBAND MUMBLE, OR AM I GOING DEAF?

Under the category of things I wish I knew when I was younger is that we actually need to protect our ears. Hearing loss can be inherited or acquired from illness, but it can also come from too much exposure to loud noise. My friend Wendy recently told me that her doctor recommends seeing an audiologist in our forties to get a baseline test, but so far I'm in denial. My cousin tells me she wears earplugs when she blow-dries her hair, and going forward I'm going to start wearing them at SoulCycle.

Another close friend, Rachel, recently reported that she's developed ringing in the ears, otherwise known as tinnitus. It sounds like living hell! She hears continuous buzzing in her ears, and it's particularly loud when she's trying to fall asleep. Can you imagine?! And this is very common, affecting an estimated 50 million adults in the United States. For most people, it's an annoyance that they can adjust to, but in severe cases tinnitus can cause people to have difficulty concentrating and sleeping, as you can imagine. The only good news about these hearing issues is that they are *not* caused by estrogen depletion; this is just plain old aging.

All this is hard stuff and is also just life. The one thing I know for sure that won't cure health problems is denial, so my core message on the health front is don't put your head in the sand—don't miss those doctor's appointments, pay attention to changes in how you feel and look, and talk to your friends about things that worry you. I've learned so much about my body from the Woolfers, from discovering that dark brown perimenopausal vaginal sludge is actually normal (hard to imagine, it's so revolting, like dragon's blood) to being reminded to get a bone-density scan. The power of shared knowledge and communication is huge and can be lifesaving!

CHAPTER EIGHT

(WORK AND MONEY)

BUT HOW WILL I PAY FOR MY DEPENDS?

Take your life in your own hands, and what happens?
A terrible thing: no one to blame.

—ERICA JONG

I FIND THAT ALMOST ANY discussion of career and finances at this point in our lives can be emotionally laden. The harsh reality is that, as with many other things—perky breasts, lustrous hair, and small children (if we had them)—our best earning years are very possibly behind us, and the choices and mistakes we made along the way have shaped our financial reality. Most of us are grappling with accepting where we are, wondering what we can still contribute and achieve, while also, as one friend puts it (making arms like a marine crawling under barbed wire six inches off the ground as she says this), "crawling to the finish line" as we start to contemplate retirement.

When it comes to work, by midlife most of us have friends all over the "ladder of success." I have girlfriends who stopped working when they had kids and never went back, and friends whose careers never took a pause and are now at the top of their game, running companies or their own creative agencies or working as partners at big law firms. But when I look around, the majority of women I know are somewhere in between, like myself actually. They've had some career success, whether big or small, and some failure, some left turns, and sometimes years of stumbling. Many are on second or third careers, sometimes by design, but more often it just sort of happened.

A moving thread started by an anonymous Woolfer highlighted the melancholy and complications that so many of us feel around money and career at midlife:

> I consider myself a feminist. However, I made choices in my life that led me to become financially dependent upon my husband. After getting married, I put my career on hold and worked part-time in my field (arts administration) for fifteen years while my kids were growing up. The work was interesting, but my career did not progress. I had the option to do these things because my husband did well enough to support us and even afford luxuries like private school and a second home. I am now in my early 50s and have my own business. I am still not making a lot of money and I am disappointed in myself that I can't contribute more to the expenses. Lately my husband holds it over my head that he is the breadwinner. I feel that despite a good marriage, there is definitely a power imbalance due to the income imbalance. My kids are also aware

that he pays for our lifestyle. I started out by saying that I am a feminist, but sometimes I feel like a fraud. While I loved raising my kids and it was incredibly important to me, I do regret not achieving more in the world. Does anyone else feel like this?

SUSAN: You are definitely not alone. What upsets me the most is how much we as a society equate financial gain with being a valuable, productive member of society.

REBECCA: Oh, honey, we're the same age, and I took the other path. I didn't stay home with my son, I put him in childcare and went back to work, and I actually out-earned my husband last year. But it doesn't affect the personal dynamic; I consider myself a feminist, but in the house I'm still "the wife."

EMILY: Yes, I have definitely felt like a fraud at times and wondered often what I might have achieved if I had done things differently. You are so not alone. And I encourage my daughters to be independent and not rely on men to support them!

ROBIN: 1/ you're still a feminist; 2/ feeling like a fraud or failure is normal but shouldn't be confused with actually being a fraud or a failure; 3/ I know a lot of people our age (men too) taking stock and realizing they have underachieved or never intended to be dependent; 4/ we can always regret our choices. It's just a sign that we are learning more about our values or needs. And it's never too late for a reset or realignment.

JENNY: I tend to side with Carlos Castaneda, who observed: "All paths lead nowhere," and "the question to ask ourselves is: does this path have a heart?" It sounds, Anonymous, like you chose (as I did, and continue to, because it's the only way I know) a path with heart, with all the mess and lack of approval that sometimes accompanies it. Don't abandon this ethos now, and don't abandon your heart. Exciting new chapters await.

I adore the loving hopefulness of Jenny's "all paths lead nowhere" comment, and to know Jenny personally is to know one of the warmest and most optimistic women around. I tend to be a little darker, though, and now, around fifty, like Anonymous and many of the women who responded to her, I look back and see alternate paths I wish I had taken. Our stories may be different, but ambivalence about one's own trajectory, career and otherwise, is a staple of middle age.

Right out of college, in the Paleolithic age, I started a career in book publishing as an entry-level literary scout for European publishers. My boss was a woman in her forties and a huge inspiration to me. She controlled her own hours and was happily pregnant, reading manuscripts in her pink-painted offices. She was such an inspiration, in fact, that three years later, when I turned twenty-three, I started my own small agency to compete with her (the very same month I was married and got pregnant myself).

Nina Collins Associates burgeoned throughout my twenties, and before long I had five employees, sixteen clients in as many foreign countries, a lease on a SoHo office, and a big-ass copy machine. I loved that business. Every Friday I would lug home, in enormous canvas totes, thousands of pages of manuscripts for my weekend reading. Come Monday I'd be ready to rumble—competing for information, managing my small (and equally young) staff, meeting with editors and agents all over the city. It was fast paced and felt glamorous; I got to use my German language skills, travel to Europe, and spend a ton of time wining and dining. I remember flitting around town in my discount Norma Kamali blazers with shoulder pads, and one particularly sexy short skirt/vest/blazer number in black from Armani that made me feel oh so sophisticated.

I was extremely ambitious in those days, fueled by the scary hole left by my mother's death and a need to prove—to myself as much as anyone else—that I could build something from scratch and support myself; that I could and would be okay in the world. I worked hard and I was okay! I had a SEP IRA, gave generous bonuses, and was earning six figures *on my own steam* well before I was thirty. It was a buzz, but I wasn't happy inside. The external flurry was masking a lot of inner turmoil, the unresolved gunk of messy beginnings.

Have you ever noticed that your best qualities can also be your worst? I think this is true of most people if you look closely. In my case, I can be extremely effective and equally impetuous. In my twenties, not so surprisingly, I was also acutely lacking in self-awareness. I wasn't always the nicest boss. I could be demanding, shrill, and totally impatient. I've always been a planner, an organizer, a woman of action, and nothing gets my adrenaline going like a good to-do list. When I cross stuff off (preferably with a black Sharpie), I get a rush of calm superiority, the way I imagine cocaine feels for some people. The downside of this nearly manic efficiency is a steamroller-like quality that emerges. I *do*, with verve, and I don't really want to listen to anyone else. I also fling myself toward change, embracing the new—learning new things, being in new environments, having the next adventure—in a way that seems beyond the norm, more than the average Jane. This makes me inspiring to some, but infuriating to others, and hard to keep up with. I'm often on to the next thing before my kids/employees/partners have time to exhale. With age and reflection, I've at least recognized these things about myself, but in my twenties I just steamrolled.

I've also realized that my almost crazed ambition during those years masked a lot of pain and depression. Or tried to cover it up, anyway. I was still grieving the loss of my mother and the chaos of my childhood. Instead of sitting down and taking a breather for some major therapy, I responded by building a very big life—young marriage, many children, big career—and ignoring what was underneath. *Go, go, go!*

I worked like a lunatic until my second pregnancy with twins at age twenty-eight landed me on bed rest, and the forced hiatus gave me an opportunity to reflect on my future. What I realized was that I didn't want to be a literary scout for the rest of my life. My decision to close up shop was not as much about wanting to stay home with my babies (as adorable as they were) as about feeling an itch to do something different. I gave my clients and staff six months' notice and shuttered a successful business. I stayed at home for two years, lived off my generous husband, had a fourth child, and read the *New York Times* every day in great detail.

At thirty-one, ready to do something else, and only knowing the publishing business, I decided to open a literary agency representing authors, this time with a (male) partner instead of being the sole head of an enterprise. Slightly older and maybe a smidge smarter, I no longer wanted to work *quite* so hard. At the same time, my marriage was foundering, I had four small children, and I was feeling increasingly depressed. I thought acting as an agent would be more creative and less reactive, and also move at a slower pace, so I could focus more on my life and family. The business worked, and for a bunch of years we chugged along, but I found myself less and less engaged, and eventually things started to fizzle. My heart was not in it, and I had the incredible good fortune to be able to rely on my then husband, as his career had begun to take off. My business partner, frustrated with standing by while my drive dwindled (the notorious drive that drew him to me in the beginning), went off on his own, right around the time my husband and I decided to get divorced. So both my marriage and my business imploded at the same time—simultaneous breakups with two men—and I found myself in a precarious emotional spot. Without putting too fine a point on it, I was thirty-eight years old and a complete wreck: the whole life around which I had formed my adult identity was flat on its ass.

I decided to step off the publishing ladder for good and went home to be with my kids and try to heal some of my wounds. During the next decade I bounced around to different projects and jobs: I started to write, went to grad school and completed a master's in narrative medicine at Columbia, got a certificate as a life coach, and for two and a half years made a short but fulfilling detour working in a hospital to create an empathy program for the residents. I kept busy, but during the years between thirty-five and forty-five I often felt anxious and wondered what the hell I was going to do with my life that had any meaning.

In the second half of my forties, I felt a shift, a coalescing of different interests and opportunities that provided me with a renewed sense of purpose. I became very involved in resurrecting the literary and film career of my late mother, and to my delight and surprise, her "lost" film, *Losing Ground*, and collection of mostly unpublished writings, *Whatever Happened to Interracial Love?*, have become critical hits. During this phase, I also remarried, started getting hot flashes, and sent all my children out into the world. These changes, along with the hundreds of sticky issues and desperate middle-of-the-night questions that accompanied them, inspired me to create the "What Would Virginia Woolf Do?" Facebook group on a lark, which led to the writing of this book you hold in your hands. I now feel like I can call myself a writer and a consultant, and my next plan is to finish that memoir I started almost ten years ago.

To sum it all up, the course of my career has been: bright, rising star in my twenties, crash and burn in my thirties, and an unexpected new path in my forties. Not that I've figured it all out, but at least I'm motivated again and I've stopped whining. After closing my second business, it was painful to feel so aimless (depression, feelings of loserdom). I fully acknowledge my privilege, that I had the freedom to get a little lost, to question, and to flounder. That freedom also extended my limbo phase and left me endlessly seeking the "right" thing. For me the jury is out on the question: is there always a "right" thing, or not?

KNOCK, KNOCK. CAN SOMEBODY PLEASE LET ME BACK IN?

IN ANY CASE. DO I HAVE career regrets? Yes. As grateful as I am that I was able to make the choice in my late thirties to step off the hamster wheel, and while I appreciate the many experiences that I may not have ever had if I'd stuck it out being an agent, if you put a gun to my head right now and asked me to choose, I'd say I regret dropping out of my publishing career. I spent eighteen years building something, and I walked away. I think I'd feel pretty damn proud of myself if I had stayed and grown that business and made it really work for the long haul. Most women I know who stopped working mid-career feel that way. Woolfer Beverly, a writer on her fourth career, said to me while reflecting on her own path, "It's difficult to know how much a job can shape the tone and meaning of one's day." And I so agree. A job gives us an independent identity, a sense of purpose, tangible praise and rewards. It's not so easy to re-create that through caregiving, volunteer work, taking care of a home, or hobbies. I think about the housewives of previous generations who might have been master gardeners, PTA chairs, expert seamstresses, virtuosic musicians, but still felt "less than" their working husbands.

And then there's the money. There's no denying that having your own money—earning it, saving it, controlling how it's spent—is essential in terms of feeling agency and power in your life. I'm not saying at all that it's "bad" to depend on anyone financially. There may be a million reasons to do that, including just wanting to, but every woman should have her eyes wide open about the trade-offs she's making when it comes to money and work.

It can be infantilizing for a grown woman to have to ask her partner for cash, and I know of husbands who dissect their wives' credit card bills while their own spending is opaque. This can lead to messed-up behavior like shoplifting "little luxuries" or slipping a couple of twenties out of a wallet that was left on the top of a bureau. More problematic is when the breadwinner dies and the spouse left behind, who assumed everything was taken care of, discovers the life insurance has expired or there's a secret pile of debt. The financial imbalance doesn't always bring out the best in people.

That said, the majority of women ages twenty-five to fifty-five are employed (about 70 percent, according to the Organization for Economic Cooperation and Development), and my friends who never left the work world seem overall to be glad they stayed, even though they went through some tough times along the way. Woolfer Kara, a corporate lawyer at a fancy New York City firm, says, "I had to stay in the game when I had my kids because my husband and I really couldn't afford to stay in the city on just his salary. I had my kids fairly early on in my career (midthirties, but still a baby lawyer) and it was tough. Many an episode of crying in the shower and feeling pulled between two inexhaustible demands—that of my children and that of my job. However, over time, the kids got older, and I got more senior. It didn't get necessarily easier (I still work as hard), but it got somehow more manageable. On balance, I am really glad that I stuck with it as it has afforded me a career that would be hard, if not impossible, to re-create had I taken those years off…"

It can feel like a huge gift and privilege if you can afford to quit work for a while and stay at home, particularly when you are young and fresh and there's so much to do with managing home, children, and relationships. But as we age, and no longer feel as much value placed on our roles as mothers and new wives, work can be a great source of confidence and identity. Without it, we can flounder, feel more invisible, feel we have less to offer, and all that can be brutal to self-esteem, which then hurts us in all areas of our lives.

Nothing in life has an expiration date. You are free to change at any age.

—MAIRA KALMAN

Women who were building their careers in their twenties or thirties and opted out for five, ten, or more years to raise children (or play tennis, or volunteer, or spend a lot of time in therapy) usually find that it's not so easy to jump back in, and certainly not at the salary they would have been making had they "leaned in" and stuck it out. (An infuriating side note: even the most qualified and highest educated "leaners" lose 10 percent of their potential earnings *per* child.) For one thing, the technological savvy required by most white-collar jobs has changed radically. Some positions require a social media presence even to get in the door; try starting up a new Twitter account in your forties and see how many followers you get aside from your niece Mary and the stalkerish guy at Spin class. You know how we're always asking our kids to program the DVR or navigate a new iTunes interface after an automatic update? That's how my friend Denise feels when she asks her twenty-four-year-old colleagues to explain (over and over) the content management system she needs to create copy in her new job with an online clothing retailer. Meanwhile, she's forty-eight and her manager is twenty years her junior. "I really try to avoid letting my colleagues know my age," she says. "If they do find out, they either act like I've passed gas in the hallway or treat me like their mother and corner me in tears after an awful Tinder date."

"I think women underestimate how hard it is to get back into the game," observed Woolfer Carla. Age discrimination may be illegal, but according to a survey by AARP, about 20 percent of job seekers over forty-five believe that they didn't get hired for a particular position because they were considered too old. Another study published in 2017 by the Federal Reserve Bank of San Francisco found "compelling evidence" that older people, and especially women, experience age discrimination in hiring (and, of course, the same discrimination applies to people who have lost their jobs and are seeking new ones, not just those who opted out for a time). The researchers created more than forty thousand fake résumés that were identical except for age and gender and submitted them online for more than thirteen thousand mostly lower-skilled jobs. They found that response rates went down as age went up, and the disparity was significantly higher for women than for men. The report comes when the percentage of the U.S. adult population age sixty-five and older is projected to rise sharply, which will increase the ratio of nonworkers to workers and strain the Social Security system.

Let's hope that studies like this will affect public policy and things will change, but let's also not hold our breath. In the meantime, it's common for career counselors to advise point blank, "Dye your hair and bleach your teeth." A recent article in *Forbes* suggested beauty and fashion tips that could help women "shave years off their age" for a job interview. Translation: the real you is too old. According to economist Joanna Lahey, an expert on age and sex discrimination, the bias against hiring older women begins as early as thirty-five!

My friend Marina has a classic tale along these lines. Marina is a lanky, gorgeous former college athlete who stepped out of her promising career in advertising a few years after she married an equally promising (male) colleague and they started having children. As the kids grew into adolescence Marina got restless and started wanting back into the game, but she found it really hard. The exploration she describes led her down all sorts of "goofy paths including lifeguarding, a suicide hotline, and after-school homework helper," before eventually landing in real estate. And very fortunate timing too, because right around the time she got her license, her husband was diagnosed with Parkinson's and is now unable to work.

Marina loved staying home with her kids, but was it worth it? "The journey getting back in was humiliating," she says. Now her kids are almost out of college and her husband is at home. Jen is the breadwinner and she's feeling very proud of herself as she pays the last dregs of tuition and cares for her partner. She reports, "It will be five years in October. I feel part of the world now. I feel better about myself and even look and dress better. I'm more respected by my peers and admired by my family. Now my biggest problem is that I'm working too hard! It's like giving a thirsty person a glass of water."

If you are struggling to get a job after a stint out of the workplace or to keep working when you have kids, there are a number of career counseling services especially geared toward women that can help. Two companies with good reputations are Après and Path Forward. The Second Shift is a job-hunting community whose mission is to keep women with professional skills in the workforce by matching them with jobs that allow some flexibility, and Encore is an incredible nonprofit that focuses on helping people create "second-act" careers that have social impact.

BOSS BARBIE, OR WHY ARE ALL CEOS BLOND?

You know who is getting high-powered jobs? Blondes. According to research presented at the 2016 annual meeting of the Academy of Management, an international association of organization and management scholars, while just 2 percent of the world's population and 5 percent of white people in the United States have blond hair, 35 percent of female U.S. senators and 48 percent of female CEOs at S&P

500 companies are blond. Female university presidents are more likely to be blond too. Given the staying power of the "dumb blonde" stereotype, you might find this counterintuitive, but in fact, it plays right into it. Coauthor of the study Jennifer Berdahl suggests the following reasons for these blonde versus blonde discrepancies on her blog:

> Our data suggest that blonde women are not only assumed to be younger than their darker haired counterparts, but are also judged to be less independent-minded and less willing take a stand than other women and [also] men. In other words, Barbie can be CEO as long as she is young and/or docile, or being blonde might allow her to be older and more forceful than she otherwise could be.

A related study published in the journal *Psychological Science* about race and male Fortune 500 CEOs also caught my eye: black CEOs are more likely to have nonthreatening "teddy bear" faces (babyish round cheeks, small noses, high foreheads), while their white counterparts are less likely to have those sort of cherubic features and instead are prized for looking mean or angry.

At the time of the Women's March following the inauguration of 2017, a photo of a seventysomething woman carrying a handmade sign circulated widely. It read: "I can't believe I still have to protest this fucking shit." Yep.

RESET BUTTON, ANYONE?

REINVENTION MIGHT BE a cliché of middle age, but it's reality for many. Whether by necessity (death, divorce) or choice, it's common for Americans today to have two or three or even four career paths in their lives. According to the *Wall Street Journal*, between the ages eighteen and forty-two most workers have had upward of ten different jobs. But starting over is also harder as we get older, and particularly so if you are feeling faded and less attractive on the job market to employers, not to mention daunted by the business world's youth culture. (I have trouble with Excel; forget Instagram.)

It's not just women who stepped out of the workforce. I have a college friend who seemed to have the most exciting career. While I was on a circuitous path that included some successes, motherhood, some failures, and attempts at reinvention, she moved in a consistent upward trajectory from small-town reporter to nightly news producer to an executive making documentary films. She won awards, traveled the world, bought herself a lovely Victorian house in San Francisco. We see each other about once a year, and over the past few years, she says the only thing that motivates her anymore is trying to earn enough money to cash out and move somewhere cheaper like Costa Rica. Because of video streaming and the Internet, the industry has radically changed and it's hard to make money and not a whole lot of fun anymore. Like a number of women (and men) I know who had been successful for decades in fields like photography, graphic design, magazines, and book publishing, she's wondering how to remake herself at fiftysomething and earn enough to retire.

That said, stories abound—I like to think of them as *More* magazine–type stories—of real women who have gripped life by the balls and forged a new path. And they are there if you look or ask or scratch the surface. A 2017 *New York Times* article told the story of

Laura Callens, a fifty-two-year-old school admissions director who wanted to do something more personally meaningful in the wake of her husband's death. She went back to school and became a nurse and now works in the ward where he passed. Reading this article brought tears to my eyes (the courage! the science! GREs at fifty-two!) and prompted me to ask in the group what Woolfers thought about re-invention. No surprise, they're all over it:

> **CARLA:** I have a friend who worked in tech, and at fifty, switched to teaching math in NYC and then won a major award for her work teaching international students.

> **JENNIFER:** I became a financial adviser at forty-four and it's my third and hopefully final career. First I was a television and radio producer; then I was a fundraiser/nonprofit executive.

> **MATTIE:** My sister-in-law went back to school to become a P.A. in emergency medicine. So brave.

> **BETSY:** I got my first dot-com job, as an information architect, when I was fifty-five.

> **CHERIE:** I'll be fifty when I start a PhD program this fall. Why not? I will be fifty-six in six years whether I do it or not.

STEPHANIE: Love this story, and stories like it— which are almost always about women. I became a corporate communications person at age fifty, after years in the restaurant business and stay-at-home-momming. I became a novelist at age sixty. This year, at sixty-one, I became a writing workshop teacher and I'm working on novel number two and personal essays. I've gone back to drawing classes, an early love. I have daily challenges to overcome or tiptoe around or bump into to pursue my passions, and I wish it were easier but it is so worth it.

It's inspiring, but let's not kid ourselves: sometimes there aren't many options and we have to stick with jobs we hate in order to pay the bills. Or we can't find a job or are living on public assistance, barely getting by. Here's a pet peeve of mine. How many times have you heard versions of these two career-related maxims? "Reinvention is always an option" and "It's essential to find your passion." As hopeful as they sound, these notions can also be mythical traps (and they are certainly luxuries of privilege). My friend Lucinda is a literary agent who would love to switch gears and find another career, but at fifty-five with a kid to raise and virtually no savings after a financially devastating divorce, reinvention doesn't seem all that possible. And the "finding your passion" bit? Most people can't make a living running marathons or baking pies or knitting or reading Victorian novels. I suppose some can, but let's be real: 99 percent can't, and it feels downright demoralizing to be told that you're not fulfilled because you haven't "found your passion."

There's taking account of where we are—the reality of midlife crisis—juxtaposed with the reality of financial planning: what we can and should do to be smart about our financial futures. The core message, really the only message here from me, is *take ownership of your choices and take responsibility for your own finances.* It's crucial. The fantasy that the world (or your parents, partner, or children) will take care of you is just that, a fantasy. They may all help, and I hope they do, but in the end *you* need to take care of *you.*

LET'S GET REAL: THE NITTY-GRITTY OF FINANCIAL PLANNING

RUTH: I want to reinvent myself as retired.

I KNOW MORE THAN ONE (in fact, I can think of at least five, and those are just the ones who have admitted it to me) smart, capable woman who has no idea how much the monthly mortgage payment is, or whether and how much life insurance their partner has, or where the policies might be, or if they are even in effect. I think this is a huge mistake, and it's a lesson I learned when I was nine. My mother's only sister, Francine, who lived in Rochester and was married to a Xerox executive, found out one day that he was leaving her for his secretary. Francine was a stay-at-home mom with three kids, a station wagon, and a dog, and she didn't even know where the checkbook was kept, not to mention how to use it. My grandmother came to stay with me and my brother while my mom went up to Rochester for two whole weeks to coach her sister in the business of life. It left an impression. Whether you're married, single, or divorced, there are some absolute basics—the fiscal equivalent of being aware of your cholesterol levels and blood pressure and getting regular Pap smears and mammograms—that every woman should know and do.

New York City accountant Shelly Jacobson Taylor, EA, CPA, agrees and underscored the pitfalls of this kind of fiscal ignorance to me. "What I often see, especially when women are going through a divorce, is that they don't have a clue about the family finances." She added, "If anything goes wrong such as death or divorce, they are often blindsided. Sometimes they discover that they have been living beyond their means, and there is a lot of debt that they weren't aware of."

Our attitudes about finances—whether we are frugal or profligate, whether we wake up at four a.m. anxious about the gas bill or never know our bank balance and feel totally relaxed about that—come from deep places and often go back to childhood. I was raised by a strong mother, but she was an artist, so we were really quite poor (all my clothes until I was at least thirteen came from the thrift shop, for example), and she and my father were divorced and fought about money constantly. Hence, I have two core beliefs around money: (1) an anxiety that I won't have enough and (2) a feeling of competence that I can deal with that, whatever comes. I'm grateful for the latter.

Because my mother was forceful and capable and always managed to pay the bills and take care of my brother and me, in my gut I know I can do the same. Yes, I worry when I have lots of big expenses, and in my perfect fantasy world of course I wish someone else could just take care of everything. Who wouldn't want that, really? The pressure and tedium and relentless quality of the business of life sucks. But giving it all over to someone else is a fantasy I don't entertain seriously, because it's not an objectively smart way for anyone to live. During my first marriage, my husband managed our finances (he was fifteen years older, worked in finance, and made more money, so that division of labor seemed sensible), but I still felt the need to know the ins and outs of what was going on, so much so that I eventually wound up taking over paying the daily bills, which forced me to ask questions, which led to me learning about his business. It was all very useful and informative, particularly when we were on opposite sides of the table ending our marriage. Keeping my head in the sand about our financial situation was never something I felt comfortable doing, and, damn, am I happy I inherited this particular trait from my mother.

Why? I'm sure you know why even if it's extremely unpleasant to think about: death, divorce, illness, injury, job loss. These are events that happen all the time, are often unexpected, and too frequently leave financial hardship in their wake.

If you feel ashamed about your ignorance, consider this to be a proverbial judgment-free zone. You may have missed the boat on a great investment or real estate deal in the past, but there are steps you can take right now to help protect your future.

MONEY MATTERS

*DANA: Does raising my girls to take care of me in my old age
count as a retirement plan?*

LOL. BUT SERIOUSLY, how do you save money?

A report by the Economic Policy Institute, an independent non-profit think tank that researches the impact of economic trends and policies on working people in the United States, states that "nearly half of families have no retirement-account savings at all," and according to the Fidelity Investments Retirement Savings Assessment, 55 percent of American households risk not being able to cover essential expenses like housing, health care, and food in retirement.

It happens; time flies. Maybe we never earned enough to feel like we could sock away any extra cash, or maybe, like a few close friends, we suffered significant financial loss after a divorce. Or maybe we were reckless and spent like there was no tomorrow, wasting money on shoes and gin and travel, thinking that old age would never come. Wherever you are on this continuum, by age fifty, the specter of retirement is looming, and we'd be fools not to be wondering how we are going to afford it.

One of the biggest conundrums here, of course, is simply that we are living longer. By sixty, some of us may feel we have enough money saved in our retirement accounts to last another ten or fifteen years, but we know from the actuarial tables that we could easily live another twenty. Who's going to pay for that?! The sixty-five-year retirement age for Social Security was established in 1933, when a typical retirement lasted eight to ten years. Fast-forward to today, and longevity has increased, so the new reality is that we have to work longer or save more, or both.

Friend and financial coach Amanda Clayman tells me, "If you're not a natural saver, then saving is a muscle you can build." CPA Jacobsen adds that there are so many temptations to overspend, which can hijack your savings—and credit cards add to the problem. "Women often go very *Gone with the Wind* when they're shopping with credit cards," she says. "In other words, they 'will think about it tomorrow.'" She suggests that we start paying for things in cash. "People often are much more willing to turn over a credit card than they are to give up the cold, hard cash." She also makes the great point that if you can't live on what you are earning when you are working, how are you going to be able to survive in retirement?

Once you have your debt paid off and are able to save, my financially savvy friends recommend Fidelity and Vanguard as low- or no-fee places to get started with investing and saving. One bit of brass-tacks advice is to go to the Social Security Administration and figure out what you will be receiving. Then use a retirement calculator to figure out what you can expect to see from your current assets (Moneychimp has one). From there, you can start to construct a plan. Clayman's tips include building an emergency fund and setting a financial goal and working toward it; sometimes hitting small goals increases motivation. She also points out that when we're inexperienced in an area, we're often afraid to make mistakes. Ask others, read books, interview prospective financial advisers. Some of the books I've personally found useful are Jan Cullinane's *The Single Woman's Guide to Retirement* (because even if you aren't single, it's often helpful to think as if you are), Tony Robbins's *Money: Master the Game*, and the James B. Stewart classic, *Den of Thieves*.

ANDREA: *My advice would be to take care of yourself. First and foremost. Don't rely on other people to do it. They won't always be there. And you deserve it. You deserve to be independent.*

IT'S COMPLICATED: DIVORCE, SECOND MARRIAGES, STEPKIDS, PRENUPS

I'VE BEEN DIVORCED AND REMARRIED; I've had stepchildren and also a prenuptial agreement. So while there are a million different ways to approach these things, I do speak from experience. What I can say is that all of the above is heart-wrenchingly complicated—obviously emotionally, but also from a straightforward financial point of view, which is what I'll briefly tackle here.

Divorce costs everyone a lot of money. There's no way around this reality. I'll make it very simple: there's a pie, and it's going to get cut, basically in half. One household is going to become two, and that's more expensive, and each partner will be running it with less money. One of my closest friends, whom I'll call Samantha, was completely brought to her knees by her divorce. She was in her forties and the primary breadwinner (by far), and her husband really enjoyed being a stay-at-home dad, so much so that he fought her tooth and nail in the divorce. All the legal bills were on her, and he fought so hard that they wound up paying for things like forensic accountants and court-appointed guardians, all of which added up to a staggering bill in the hundreds of thousands of dollars. What could have been a straight-forward divorce, even something that could have been easily medi-ated (modest assets, one kid), forced her to sell her house and cleaned out her retirement accounts. She ended up living in a rental apart-ment and using food stamps while she got back on her feet. Almost five years later, and now over fifty, she's now financially where she was when she was thirty.

That's not an uncommon story, so plan and think carefully before you divorce, and think hard about how you'll do it. Avoid litigation at all costs if you can. Know what the assets are. Try to be fair and rational when it comes to the money. Pray your ex-partner will do the same. Then, if you are so fortunate to make it out alive and still have some money in the bank, when you go to remarry, you need to con-sider how to preserve your assets for your children, because they are not the offspring of hubby number two and they need to be protected. It's not romantic, but neither is poverty.

Any expert will tell you that the biggest pitfalls in remarriage are money and stepchildren. In fact, while the divorce rate for first mar-riages is typically reported to be around 40 to 50 percent, the stan-dard rate for second marriages tends to be in the 60 to 70 percent range. There are surely lots of reasons for this, including the realiza-tion that there is life after divorce, but to my mind much of it is related to the complications of coming together later in life, when habits and rituals are deeply grooved, histories are separate and unknown to the other, and money and children are not shared. All these things make it harder to start fresh with someone. You're not in Kansas (or twenty-five) anymore.

That said, we persist! People like to fall in love; we like the companionship, the regular sex, the travel buddy, the having a person to tell all our secrets. So I say go ahead and good luck, but make sure you have a prenup.

Even if you haven't experienced prenup stress in real life, you can probably understand why it seems like a bad word. It's not very sexy to get a legal document drawn up that spells out the financial dissolution of your union in the event of death or divorce. I get that. But the way to think about it is simple when you're old like me: it's for the children. It's not about him or you. It's about the kids. Think of it like this:

Sally is retired. She has three kids from two different marriages and sizable assets from thirty years of working and from her two divorce settlements. She wants to marry Bob, who's almost sixty and has a small accounting firm, two kids of his own, and a bit of debt, both to the IRS and to his ex-wife. This is a messy situation, and if they don't hash it out, it will be a nightmare. Who's paying what for which kids? Who owns what? What happens if Sally gets hit by a bus? What happens if in five years they are still married and Bob wants to retire but still has a lot of debt? I think you get my point. These things are not insurmountable, but they are issues—serious ones that won't go away, and if Sally and Bob have a chance in hell of staying married, they need to talk about them and get some legal advice.

Stepchildren are something that should get easier as we get older. (Finally! Something!) Hopefully they are at least almost grown-up, and you can just be a nice person in their lives and they in yours. The most optimistic way of looking at it is that life is richer with more people in it. The less rosy side, which I've also observed to be true, is that no one will ever love or know your children the way their biological parents do, so this is a stumbling block in most second and third and fourth marriages. It just is. But as we age, it becomes less of a problem. I have one friend, Wendy, who has known her stepdaughter since the girl, whom we'll call Rebecca, was six. Wendy went on to have two daughters of her own, and Rebecca had her own mother, and her time growing up was spent between the two households. The situation was a pretty good one as far as these things go, but not great, with the usual tensions of divorce and remarriage and broken families. Rebecca tolerated Wendy and Wendy did her best to love this child who was not her own (always a challenge, no matter what anyone tells you). Today, Rebecca is thirty, married, and living in another state and just had her second child, whom Wendy adores! Wendy, now fifty-five, has known and cared about Rebecca for most of her life and is now genuinely thrilled to call this new grandchild her own. It's very sweet to see and makes perfect sense. The pieces can be complicated, but they can also come together, given time and love and tolerance.

ESTATE PLANNING, LONG-TERM CARE, LIFE INSURANCE, AND WILLS

AS A REASONABLY INTELLIGENT WOMAN, I am embarrassed to report that I find aspects of estate planning (Crummey letters? trusts? all ugh) more complicated than advanced calculus. I really don't understand a lot of it when it gets very complex, and the laws change all the time. Maybe part of it is denial and the reluctance to spend so much time in the world of "when I'm dead, XYZ." But I can tell you I'm less in denial than most, and on the basics, which are so important, I'm a total stickler:

1. If you have kids, you need life insurance. I buy **term**, which is the simple kind that expires, usually after age sixty-five, or certainly by age seventy, and pays out only if death occurs during the term of the policy. By the time I'm sixty-five, my kids should be able to take care of themselves, and I will have hopefully done enough estate planning that I'm no longer quite as worried about estate taxes. But for now, I have a policy that should cover all my estate taxes and then some.

   The more complicated kind is called **whole-life**, which is a type of permanent insurance, combining life coverage with an investment fund. Here you're buying a policy that pays a stated, fixed amount on your death, and part of your premium goes toward building cash value from investments made by the insurance company.

Consult a professional for advice here. Among the many things I don't understand is that many financially savvy people seem to frown on whole-life, even though it sounds like the better option. Do what's right for you and your family, but have life insurance if there's anyone you could leave behind who depends on you.

2. Everyone should have a will! Everyone! I am dumbfounded by the number of friends I have who don't have one. Take it from me, please. When my mother died without a will, it caused so much unnecessary and expensive pain that was completely avoidable. Not only should you have a will, but you should revisit it every five years or so, because things change (your assets, your priorities, your children's stage of life and their needs, your philanthropic interests, federal laws), and you don't even realize how much until you are forced to sit down and think about it. Health care proxies and living wills should be part of this process, and it's all really not that hard, I promise you. A simple will can be a simple experience and you can even do it online, although I recommend finding a nice, reasonable lawyer and having an actual conversation about estate planning at least a few times during your later adulthood. The guy I use was a Match.com date. I didn't want to sleep with him, but he only charged me $2,500 for a complete estate-planning overhaul, and now he gets my referrals!

3. My last tip is sort of dorky, and it definitely comes from someone who was caught way off guard by death: keep a document somewhere handy (but safe!)—even give it to someone you love— with instructions that detail all the main "business" of your life.

- Where all your bank accounts are, with account numbers
- Passwords to at least your major accounts, such as email, bank accounts, credit cards, and the like
- The combination to your safe, if you have one
- A list of your main financial assets
- The name and contact information for your estate lawyer, accountant, financial adviser, banker, whatever
- Details on any debt you may have

Think about what information you'd want your kids or siblings or partner to have easy access to if you were to drop dead tomorrow, and write it up. I gave my list to my brother. You can't think of everything, of course; he could get hit by a bus first and I could forget to reassign the list and then I could get hit by a bus. Nothing's perfect. But it's well-intentioned and it's also a good exercise in order and organization. Leaving people with a big mess on top of the pain of losing you isn't a loving thing to do.

LONG-TERM-CARE INSURANCE

If there was ever a sexy topic, this has to be it (not). It's awful to think about our loved ones or ourselves in a nursing home or adult day care. My friend Liz loves to quote her elderly mom, saying, "All I have to do is stay healthy and die soon." Of course, she did neither, Liz says with a sigh. Long-term-care insurance is something about which we should all, at the very least, be well-informed.

If you aren't familiar with the term, LTC insurance is coverage that provides nursing-home care, home-health care, or personal or adult day care for people over sixty-five or with a chronic or disabling condition that needs constant supervision. As Americans are living longer, with Alzheimer's on the rise, and medical technology is able to keep us alive in conditions under which we might actually prefer to be dead, the reality is that a great many of us are likely to need long-term care at the end of our lives, and perhaps equally likely to be unable to pay for it.

Unlike life insurance, which many people at least consider buying if they can afford it, especially when they have children, LTC insurance is something nobody actually wants to buy. There are no two ways about it: planning out how to pay for someone to change your diapers and wipe the drool off your chin when you can no longer feed yourself or your speech is incomprehensible is totally grim. I admit that I have not taken this step yet. But as Woolfer Marlene points out:

> It's a worry wondering how we might afford our old age...I wish I knew about LTC insurance years ago...the younger you are when you first buy it, the cheaper it is.

Denial is a powerful thing, but check out these sobering statistics provided by a 2012 report by the independent investment management and research firm Morningstar:

- **37 million:** The number of Americans age sixty-five or older in 2005
- **81 million:** The expected number of Americans age sixty-five or older in 2050
- **79:** The average age upon admittance to a nursing home
- **40 percent:** The percentage of individuals who reach age sixty-five who will enter a nursing home during their lifetimes

- **68 percent:** The probability that an individual over age sixty-five will become cognitively impaired or unable to complete at least two "activities of daily living"—including dressing, bathing, or eating—over his or her lifetime
- **10 percent:** The percentage of people who enter a nursing home who will stay there for five or more years
- **$162,425:** The annual cost of nursing-home care in Manhattan, New York
- **$60,773:** The annual cost of nursing-home care in Des Moines, Iowa—same as college!
- **$86,140:** The annual cost of nursing-home care in Tampa, Florida

I leave you with this: think about it and talk to your partner if you have one. Consider your end-of-life experiences with your parents or grandparents and the ways in which you might like your own end of life to go differently.

REGRETS, I'VE HAD A FEW: THINGS WE WOULD TELL OUR REAL OR IMAGINED CHILDREN

MONEY AND CAREER ARE AREAS where lots of us suffer from feelings of regret. "I should have saved more." "I shouldn't have left that job." "I wish I'd had more success at X." At forty, fifty, or sixty, does it help to look back on the mistakes we made, the things we wish we'd handled differently?

Yes. Making peace with what we regret is part of taking stock and moving ahead with clarity. We can't fix all the screwups, but we can try to understand them, forgive ourselves, and do things differently going forward. Renowned psychologist Erik Erikson's eighth stage of psychosocial development is what he termed "ego integrity vs. despair." The idea is that, toward the end of our lives, achieving a sense of integrity means fully accepting oneself and coming to terms with the life one has led. Accepting responsibility and coming to a sense of satisfaction with the self is essential, and failure to do so will result in a feeling of despair.

This is also an opportunity to applaud what we've done well.

Someone posted in the group, asking for business advice to give her college-age daughter as she sets out into the world, and the advice, all of it wise, was striking to me in the most common theme: save, have your own money, focus on your own choices. Here's what we would share with our daughters (and sons):

> **KATRIN:** Don't rush through life. Don't always be looking ahead and planning everything. Also, learn that you are responsible for your own happiness.

> **ILENE:** Max out on 401(k)/IRA; invest in index funds with low load, do not touch them no matter how bumpy the market. The magic of compounding is spectacular.

> **KATY:** Have a passion no one can take away from you—and be able to support yourself. If they are the same—all the better. Find a community built not only

on friends but on something that is your own and will sustain you. Have a prenup—always.

DANA: Take care of yourself. You get ONE spine, one body of skin, one set of feet…don't take them for granted or let bad habits ruin them. Heels, makeup, standing for hours at a time…they all take their toll.

DEIDRE: STAY OUT OF DEBT—even if it means missing out on some fun. You'll be older before you know it, and you can't count on making enough to pay off your debt and live a comfortable lifestyle, and nothing is worse than having debt hanging over you for years. It can keep you in relationships/jobs/living situations you want to get out of, and it's a massive weight that will affect every aspect of your life.

JENNY: If I could go back in time, I'd tell twenty-two-year-old me to worry less, experiment more, and not be afraid to follow my gut. (I do all of those things now, but it took me forever to realize I could!)

RUTHANNE: When choosing jobs always ask: 1) are there people (and at least one person I will be working closely with) here that I can learn from; 2) will this job open more doors than it closes for future opportunities. No to either question means don't take the job.

GWEN: Find a course of study you love to lead to a career you love. Always keep a separate bank account and credit card (not store credit cards, but Visa, MasterCard, Discover, American Express) in your own name. Travel whenever you can. Always stand up for what you believe. And finally, get a hobby, something you want to do just because it makes you happy.

STEPHANIE: Build your network and cultivate it. I've never gotten a job/opportunity from a want ad or a web posting.

ERIN: Buy a piece of real estate. I know a fair number of people who all made different choices as far as career, family, etc. The ones who made real estate purchases early are still doing fine, whether they are crazy artists, moms, wives, or career women. Those other things matter, it's just that real estate matters more, on a totally different league level.

KATY: 1. Get out of a bad relationship as soon as possible. GET OUT. Time wasted there is waste. 2. You are beautiful. Ask who is worthy of you, not who you can find. 3. What people DO tells you much more about them than words ever will. Look at their history of friendships, jobs, families.

Here are my two cents added to all this great advice: building your own business and being able to control your own schedule are the way to go in terms of lifestyle, parenting, and feeling powerful. Also, buy a piece of real estate as early as you can.

It's intense confronting aging, children growing up and moving on, and thinking about your financial future all at the same time—not to mention massive and soul-shaking existential questions like "Have I contributed something positive to life on this earth?" But if you look back with clear eyes, I know that you will see more than regret and paths not taken and realize how many skills you have accumulated along the way and how smart you are compared to your twenty- or thirtysomething self. Our choices may be limited, but unfettered from the distractions and expectations that go along with being a younger woman, this can be the ideal time to forge ahead with integrity and a more transparent understanding of what is most important to you as a person. In the words of Sheryl Sandberg, "So please ask yourself: What would I do if I weren't afraid? And then go do it."

CHAPTER NINE

(YOU'RE GONNA MAKE IT AFTER ALL)

I CREATED THE "What Would Virginia Woolf Do?" Facebook group because suddenly one September, I started waking up in the middle of the night, like clockwork, often with a pool of sweat between my breasts. I would fall asleep in the evenings normally, like I had for every night of my adult life, and then find myself eyes wide open, mind as clear as a bell, staring at the walls, from four a.m. to around six a.m. This had never happened to me before, and now, out of nowhere, it was a daily occurrence, one that led to daytime exhaustion, and ultimately, depression. When I put two and two together (the sometimes skipped and ever darkening periods, the mood swings, my age) and realized I must be embarking on "the change," I became desperate for advice and support. How long would this last? How would I function, exhausted and sweaty, in the meantime? What else was in store? My doctor offered a blasé shrug and suggested putting me on the Pill. None of my girlfriends were talking about it, but I knew there was no way in hell I was the only woman suffering in this way. I reached out to a few of my favorite ladies in a secret forum on Facebook and said, "Please, talk to me about your aging woes. I need help."

KATHRYN: *I can't run as fast as I used to and all I can conclude is that it's because of reduced hormone levels. My recipe has changed. I feel like a vegan cake—no eggs or sugar, still a cake but texturally different.*

Two years later, I remain on the perimenopausal roller coaster (just last week, doing down dog in yoga class, I noticed that my knees have gotten wrinkly!), but despite my continued and ever-surprising estrogen-starved tribulations, I'm feeling distinctly more grounded in my feelings about my aging body. I know exactly what all these crappy symptoms are, and when a new one pops up (six months ago my hair started falling out; three months ago I developed a nonstop pee urge; I didn't bleed for eight months and then my period came back with a hemorrhagic vengeance) I feel confident that (a) I'm not alone, (b) I can talk about it, and (c) if I can't find a solution, I can at least find comfort. I've also come to terms with the fact that the passage we're making isn't limited to physical symptoms, and it's been healing to grapple with the emotional piece as well.

When this all started, it was a tad demoralizing. I brooded over some questions that felt existential in scope (at least in the lugubrious gray light of four a.m.). Is my value in the world diminishing? Will I lose all sense of agency as well as sex appeal? Is my body going to fall apart overnight? Around that time, I found myself sitting across from a group of twentysomething women on the subway. They were fresh out of work and talking excitedly about the night of barhopping ahead, all bared thighs, cleavage, and shiny lipstick. I admired their lustrous hair and rose-petal skin and actually found myself thinking, "These girls are all flush with estrogen, and look at poor, sad me, headed home to watch *The Good Wife* and eat a salad!" Granted, some of my anxiety was melodramatic, but it was a panic borne out of *not knowing* and *not sharing*. Those young women *were* flush with estrogen, and I am not, but I no longer feel like this is so terribly sad. Now I understand that this is a long process, probably around a decade for most of us, so I have lots of time to get used to the transition. Now I also have "the group," as I refer to the thousands of Woolfers who have become my witty and irreverent sisterhood; women who are so alive and funny and fantastically smart that it feels impossible to doubt my (our) continued value in the world.

One of the longest longitudinal studies of its kind, the Harvard Grant and Glueck Study, which followed almost eight hundred men (ahem) for seventy-five years, found unequivocally that good relationships—more than anything else—are what keep us healthy and happy. Today the study is looking at the two thousand baby-boomer daughters and sons of the original participants and drawing the same conclusions. I'd always heard the axiom that relationships are crucial for long-term health and well-being and relied on my beloved and close circle of girlfriends to get me through hard times, but never has the power of community been more clear to me than since I developed close, intimate relationships with thousands of middle-aged female strangers through social media. I went from feeling isolated and glum, with my hot flashes and insomnia, to laughing about it online with an enormous group of brilliant and hilarious women. I wouldn't recognize 90 percent of them if I saw them at the supermarket, yet we've shared some of the most private details of our lives. I realized we were on to something very early on, when one woman posted that the group had become her best friend, and no one laughed her off the page. We get it!

One of the things that surprised me from the start is how relatively little Woolfers talk about their romantic partners or their children. For some of us, it's the first time we have felt unfettered from the immediate needs of our families and clearheaded enough to start thinking, "What's in it for me?" It's hard to convey the breadth of what we share. Whether we are debating the latest political assault on women's rights, the best literary novel to take on a long flight, the pros and cons of silicone lube, or the virtues of the Roomba, I'm constantly floored by the wisdom, humor, sex appeal, and compassion of the women who surround me. We both inspire and normalize, make one another feel badass and at the same time reassure one another that we're all okay, that everything we're feeling and experiencing is common and normal, not crazy or pathetic or old! For example, the urge to stay in bed all day:

An enormously freeing thing is to see how long you can stay in bed. Read in bed, watch TV in bed, eat in bed, sleep in bed (if you can sleep). It is wonderful to commit on, say, a Saturday, to just staying in bed.

If people ask what you are doing, say, "I'm in menopause. One of the recommended cures is bed rest." I'm serious! When you really get bored with it, you will get out of bed—eventually. But why rush it?

—SANDRA TSING LOH, *THE MADWOMAN IN THE VOLVO*

Someone posted that quote in the group and we resounded in cheerful agreement. I could practically hear the women nodding in unison through my laptop.

Kind support abounds, but there is also real-world tension and anger and disagreement. Sadly, some women have left in a huff. A thread on whether it's okay to slut shame Melania for her nudie pics was a hot potato. Another controversy was the long-married woman who posted looking for support when her secret lover of five years dumped her. Or even the time we discussed what physical indignities you most hate about getting older. Some women just don't find that shit funny. Big surprise: a bunch of grown-up, opinionated, hormonal ladies piss one another off now and then. On occasion, the defectors return, and we're so happy to have them back, and there are fabulous new women joining every day. It's not a utopia, but it's pretty darn great.

As you get older, you don't get wiser. You get irritable.

—DORIS LESSING

Be cranky, be sexy, be celibate, be whatever you want. We're entering a rather exhilarating new phase of our lives where we hopefully still have our health, but are no longer encumbered by little children, needy husbands (we've learned to claim our space), our periods, our estrogen–caregiving–child-rearing impulses, and the patriarchal tyranny of having to worry about our looks so much and try to be appealing all the time. We have lots of knowledge to share and self-knowledge to guide us. We laugh more. We don't flip out as easily. And today, more than any generation that came before us, we really are as free as men to live productive and powerfully engaged lives well into our older years.

I'm not just seeing this in the group; it's in the culture. The group just gives us a place to revel in it! Aging for women *is* changing, and in the right direction. There's less shame about our wrinkles and shifting bodies, and considerably more zest. I recently came across this truly heinous Rush Limbaugh quote from sometime during the 2016 presidential election:

> Will this country actually want to watch a woman get older before their eyes on a daily basis?

Well, yes, you asshole. Hillary Clinton actually won the popular vote and I'm pretty confident we'll have a female in the Oval Office before I hit the nursing home scene. Despite the crushing disappointment on Election Day 2016, when many of us strutted around clothed in white from head to toe, only to find ourselves, slack mouthed, in front of our TV screens at ten p.m. (I went to sleep crying that night, and I know I was not alone), we are *surrounded* these days by sheroes (female heros, for those slow on the uptake). I saw Chrissie Hynde (born in 1951) on stage in Madison Square Garden last winter and was blown away by how commanding and sexy she is. To name a small handful: Sonia Sotomayor. Ruth Bader Ginsburg. Sheryl Sandberg. Cecile Richards. Gloria Steinem. Helen Mirren. Elizabeth Warren. Joan Didion. Elena Ferrante. Jane Fonda and Lily Tomlin, both pushing eighty, and selling lube and vibrators for atrophied vaginas as characters on a popular Netflix series! Angela Merkel. Melinda Gates. Maxine Waters. Patti Smith. Martha Nussbaum. Chelsea Handler. Nicole Kidman. Anne Lamott. Viola Davis. Cora Diamond. Barbara Lee. Barbara Ehrenreich. Joan Jonas. Oprah. Anna Wintour. Mira Nair. Jane Pauley. Kathryn Bigelow. Jhumpa Lahiri. Toni Morrison. Judith Butler. Lydia Davis. Zadie Smith. Frances McDormand. Sarah Vowell. Bonnie Raitt. Billie Jean King. Marilynne Robinson. Jennifer Egan. Kathryn Chetkovich. Joyce Carol Oates. Alice Munro. Mary Karr. Laurie Anderson. Nancy Pelosi. Brené Brown. Cindy Sherman. Louise Erdrich. Madonna. Naomi Shihab Nye. Eve Ensler. Ellen DeGeneres. Julia Louis-Dreyfus. Catherine Opie. Emma Thompson. Christine Lagarde. Nathalie Arthaud. Samantha Power. Samantha Bee. Kara Walker. Alison Bechdel. Rachel Maddow. Joy Reid. Margaret Atwood. Shonda Rhimes. Bette Midler. Kirsten Gillibrand. Esther Perel. Sally Yates. Amy Poehler. Tina Fey. Mary Beard. Renée Elise Goldsberry. Roxane Gay. Diana Nyad. Lorna Simpson. Nicole Eisenman. J. K. Rowling. Lynn Nottage. Meryl Streep. Tilda Swinton. Diane Keaton. Michelle Obama! Most of these women are no longer having regular periods, and if they are, they won't be for long.

Some of our staying power is about aesthetics. "Fifty is the new thirty," blah blah blah. But it's true: advances in dermatology now allow us to keep our skin looking younger for longer, if we so choose. We can dye our hair purple and cut it short or leave it wild and gray if we want, and we have plenty of role models who do both. We can go gracefully into that Eileen Fisher night and embrace elastic waists and shawls, and even Crocs! (My friend Jodie picked up some really fab camouflage ones at T.J.Maxx last summer.) Or we can wear heels and tight jeans until the very end. Some of us put a lot of stock in staying "beautiful"—whatever that means—and others are genuinely glad to relax, to love our curvier bodies, to forgo the makeup, to feel less "visible." It's freeing to no longer feel like an object for the taking, and to be wise and so experienced. The point is that despite the inevitable backlash (Trump, trolls), we have more choice about how we want to live and to be seen than women have ever had before. We need to keep having the essential conversations to support and encourage one another in those choices.

More critical than the superficial issue of what we look like, there's more room now—if we take it—around the ways we can *talk* frankly about aging, and *experience* it. Women like Brené Brown and Oprah have helped us embrace our vulnerability and put away our shame, and it's done us a lot of good. It's no longer taboo to talk about menstruation in public (see the Thinx products advertising campaign) or vibrators (watch *Grace and Frankie*). Women like classicist Mary Beard (who famously took on her sexist detractors), model Lauren Hutton (who starred in a Calvin Klein underwear campaign at age seventy-three in 2017), and runner Kathrine Switzer (the first woman to run the Boston Marathon did it again in 2017, fifty years later, at age seventy) are all continuously paving the way for the rest of us to thrive in the process of getting older, in whatever fashion we desire.

I have more good news for you, and for the women who are bringing up the rear: tummy pooch, dry skin, and being alert to our mortality may not always be fun (and it's helpful to commiserate about the downsides), but the indisputable fact is that these issues come in tandem with an inner strength and sense of authenticity that none of us had when we were younger.

I threw a question out to the group: What are *the best things* about sliding into our fifties, sixties, and seventies? For one thing, it's a hell of a lot better than the alternative! Joking aside, over and over again, the Woolfers cried out, verbatim, "better sex" and "giving zero fucks." Some of the other responses:

> *ANDREA:* Actual confidence, as opposed to bravado.

> *NANCY:* I feel more free to give no shit and to break more rules. And I totally take things less personally. Other people's shortcomings are not about me— hooray!

> *MARLA:* Accumulated wisdom and broader perspective are allowing me to experiment and pursue ideas I couldn't have conceived of fifteen years ago.

KAREN: It's easy to get depressed about wrinkles and tummy fat, but the alternative is much worse. I've survived lymphoma. I still wish my eyelashes were as long as they once were, and my skin was wrinkle-free, but I am so happy to greet each day.

STEPHANIE: Fulfilling relationships with adult daughters I couldn't have foreseen. Friendships that have survived tests and time. I don't feel blindsided anymore, mostly. Not wasting time.

SHARON: No more complacency and confusion. Big picture starts to get into focus (what really matters?).

Fabulous, right?

Aging is a process, and I'm only forty-eight (!), so I certainly can't claim to know what's around the next bend. In this book, I've tried to bring to light some of the things that aren't discussed enough about this particular phase, the surprises that hit me as I entered perimenopause, with the conviction that honesty and straightforwardness can and should lead to diminished shame. There is nothing to be embarrassed about when it comes to getting older, and being able to laugh about it and be candid seem crucial to me. I'm grateful to have found my tribe. Join us, or start your own!

The preceding pages have covered a pile of material, from orgies to Birkenstocks to long-term-care insurance, but what are the major takeaways? Mine are as follows:

1. As I've said before, the power of choice. Most of us have more choice now than we've probably ever had in our lives, and certainly more than any generation of women before us. Embrace that, own it, use it, make it work for you. Alice Walker once famously said, "The most common way people give up their power is thinking they don't have any," and believe me, you do.

2. When I was writing this book, one of my early readers noted that I used the phrase "knowledge is power" four or five times, and she made me cut a few. Repetitive, yes, but I genuinely believe this is a concept that bears repeating. It's one of my mantras (see item 4 for my other one). Sir Francis Bacon said it in 1597, and I'm saying it today. Denial and ignorance will get you nowhere. This applies to our health (schedule those annual screenings; don't look the other way when something seems off!), our relationships (no falling asleep at the wheel there, please), and perhaps most important, our own self-reflection and awareness. Personally, I'm so sick of therapy that I sometimes want to put stones in my pockets like dear old Virginia, but I persist because I keep learning shit that's helpful, and stagnation is not an option.

3. Community is everything. "What Would Virginia Woolf Do?" is just one example of how women can band together and support one another in powerful ad hoc groups. Look at Pantsuit Nation or "Binders Full of Women Writers" on Facebook; the Women's March of 2017; the Pussyhat Project; She Writes; book clubs; quilting circles; 1970s consciousness-raising groups where

women all used mirrors to look at their labias! *Do something. Help others! Find a cause!* Social ties are just as important as exercise and quitting smoking for extending and enriching your life, and if nothing else, this whole Virginia Woolf experience has shown me, and all the Woolfers, the incredible power of the collective. In the group we've supported women with breast cancer, women getting divorced, and women starting new businesses. We launched a philanthropic arm to donate to causes close to our hearts, and we tell one another what to read, listen to, and watch on TV. Nothing is too minor to discuss (or too major), and nothing is embarrassing, and this has been invaluable.

KATE: *Hitting forty-seven in three weeks after being thrust into menopause at thirty-five and it's frankly been very daunting. But I'm so inspired by and comforted from the words of my global big sisters. Feels like the light at the end of the tunnel may in fact not be the speeding train I feared.*

---

4. Finally, acceptance. There's no time like the present, quite literally. You'll never be as young again as you are today, so please, go for it, whatever "it" is. The late, brilliant, feminist academic Carolyn Heilbrun said, "We in middle age require adventure." Damn straight we do. Whether it's becoming a political powerhouse and storming Capitol Hill, taking a younger lover, or

deciding to go for that PhD in microbiology or basket weaving, "Why do tomorrow what you can do today?" That's my second-favorite mantra!

For most of us, this perimenopause/menopause business will drag on for years. At the rate I'm going, by the time I get to the other side of it, I'll be well into my fifties, a place where no one will ever mistake me for a young woman again (not that they are really doing that now, but I hold on to my moments of delusion).

In her poignant essay "Pause," the poet Mary Ruefle describes getting to the other side—arriving—in a way that makes me feel free, happy, full of powerful grace:

> You are a woman, the ten years have passed, you love your children, you love your lover, but there are no longer any persons on earth who can stop you from being yourself—you have put your parents in the earth, you have buried the past. Of course in the meantime you have destroyed your life and it has to be completely remade and there is a great deal of grief and regret and nostalgia and all of that, but even so you are free, free to sit on the bank and throw stones and feel thankful for the few years or one or two decades left to you in which you can be yourself, even if a great many other women ended their lives, even if the reason they ended their lives is reported as having been for reasons having nothing to do with

menopause, which is thankfully behind you as you would never want to be a girl again for any reason at all, you have discovered that being invisible is the biggest secret on earth, the most wondrous gift anyone could have ever given you.

When I read that passage I imagine myself wearing linen (Eileen Fisher?) and sitting in the sun, maybe with napping grandchildren nearby and lots of girlfriends about to come over for tea or tequila. Ruefle even invokes our patron saint, Virginia Woolf, who took that next step and waded into the river with rocks in her pockets. But now we can remain on the grassy verge, tossing stones or hurling them, because we have one another.

(ACKNOWLEDGMENTS)

First and foremost, thanks to the legions of Woolfers who literally make me LOL and reflect every single day, not to mention teach me new things, solve my health and beauty problems, and tell me what to read and what to watch on TV. You have all enriched my life in the most surprising way and I am in awe of what we built together. A special shout-out to the ladies who help moderate with endless humor and wisdom: Kristen Buckley, Jenny Douglas, Stephanie Gangi, Kara Hailey, Robin Moore Lasky, Margaret Lee, Andrea Rashish, Heather Schroder, Stephanie Staal, Hannah Casey, Eileen Anne Wolter, Elena Siebert, Hillary Richard, and Diana Kane English.

Hugest of thank-yous to Sarah B. Weir, my collaborator on this book, whom I've known for more than twenty-five years and whose calm wisdom was utterly indispensable to this project. We wrote and edited and researched and did permissions together, all in a seamless flurry of enthusiasm and fun. It couldn't have been a better process and I'm grateful to you, Sarah.

Love and appreciation to another woman I've known for more than twenty-five years, my literary agent and dear friend, Heather Schroder. Heather has patiently talked through pretty much every idea and fear I've had in my adult life, and helped me see to the other side.

Thanks to my two best editors and close readers, Kamy Wicoff and Violet Fludzinski.

Gratitude to designer Bonnie Siegler, who suggested I write the book in the first place; to Jamie Raab, who bought it; and to Karen Murgolo at Grand Central Publishing, for being an awesome editor.

Thank you to Violet, Ella, Ruby, and Bruno, my four beautiful, brave, brilliant children, who have to put up with me, and for whom I'll always try to do better.

NOTES
AND RESOURCES

IN ADDITION TO RELYING ON THE RESOURCES listed below, sections of this book were vetted and corrected by a number of experts in different areas, especially those related to physical and mental health. I am extremely grateful to them for their help. They include: Dr. Jennifer Breznay, Dr. Laura Corio, Dr. Doris Day, Dr. Martin Gottlieb, Dr. Rose Ingleton, Shelly Jacobson, CPA, Dr. Debbie Magids, Dr. Karen Nelson, and Dr. Ina Ratner. Thanks also to Claire Cavanah of Babeland and Logan Levkoff for their advice on sexuality, and Alejandra Bejmar, fitness expert extraordinaire.

INTRODUCTION

A FEW BOOKS TO GET YOU IN THE MOOD:

Adichie, Chimamanda Ngozi. *We Should All Be Feminists*. Knopf, 2013.
Cusk, Rachel. *Outline*. Farrar, Straus & Giroux, 2015.
Cusk, Rachel. *Transit*. Farrar, Straus & Giroux, 2017.
Ferrante, Elena. The Neapolitan Novels series. Europa Editions.
Levine, Suzanne Braun. *50 Is the New Fifty*. Plume, 2009.
Moran, Caitlin. *How to Be a Woman*. Harper Perennial, 2011.
Solnit, Rebecca. *Men Explain Things to Me*. Haymarket, 2014.
Strayed, Cheryl. *Tiny Beautiful Things: Advice on Love and Life from Dear Sugar*. Vintage, 2012.

AND OF COURSE THESE:

Lee, Hermione. *Virginia Woolf*. Vintage, 1999.
Woolf, Virginia. *A Room of One's Own*. Mariner Books, 1989.
Woolf, Virginia. *Moments of Being*. Mariner Books, 1985.
Woolf, Virginia. *The Mrs. Dalloway Reader*. Edited by Francine Prose. Harcourt, 2003.
Woolf, Virginia. *On Being Ill*. Paris Press, 2012.
Woolf, Virginia. *To the Lighthouse*. Harcourt, 1927.

AND MY FAVORITE PODCAST, *2 DOPE QUEENS*!

https://www.wnyc.org/shows/dopequeens

At the time I was writing this book, relationship expert Esther Perel had just launched a fascinating podcast, *Where Should We Begin?* It's like being a fly on the wall during a real couple's therapy session. At a minimum, check out her brilliant TED Talks. **http://www.estherperel.com**

CHAPTER ONE

FASHION

Death by Eileen Fisher and Other Fashion Tragedies

FOOTWEAR

BIRKENSTOCK SANDALS
While writing this book, I changed my tune on these and now own a pair in fluorescent pink.
http://www.birkenstock.com/us

NO.6 CLOGS
I live in these all winter long.
https://no6store.com/collections/no-6-boots/products/
no-6-5-shearling-clog-boot-in-black-suede?

REPETTO BALLET FLATS
http://www.repetto.com/us/

LINGERIE

HANKY PANKY
My hands-down fave granny panty is the signature lace brief in black.
http://www.hankypanky.com/signature-lace-betty-brief.html

SPANX
http://www.spanx.com/

THINX
Just in case you're still getting your period.
https://www.shethinx.com/

TOWN SHOP
A New York City institution
https://www.townshop.com

SWIMWEAR AND CAFTANS

CALYPSO
Not cheap but beautiful caftans
http://www.calypsostbarth.com/

GOTTEX
http://gottex-swimwear.com

J.CREW
A surprisingly large selection of cover-ups and great sales
https://www.jcrew.com

LA BLANCA
https://www.lablancaswim.com

MALIA MILLS
Pricey but super chic
https://www.maliamills.com/

MODCLOTH
Also a good source of well-priced, funky clothing
https://www.modcloth.com/

PLUME
https://plumecollection.com/

SWIMSUITS FOR ALL
Their motto is: Perfect swimsuits no matter your age, shape, or size.
http://www.swimsuitsforall.com

CLOTHING

EILEEN FISHER
Let's be honest: we all need some Eileen Fisher in our closets.
http://www.eileenfisher.com/

LORD AND TAYLOR
Special-occasion dress mecca
https://www.lordandtaylor.com

TO READ

Garcia, Nina. *The Little Black Book of Style*. It Books, 2010.

Hyland, Veronique. "How to Get Your Body Caftan-Ready for Summer," *New York*, May 19, 2014. https://www.thecut.com/2014/05/how-to-get-your-body-caftan-ready-for-summer.html.

Karr, Mary. "High Maintenance," *The New Yorker*, May 16, 2016. http://www.newyorker.com/magazine/2016/05/16/down-with-high-heels.

Picardie, Justine. *Coco Chanel, The Legend and the Life*. It Books, 2011.

von Furstenberg, Diane. *The Woman I Wanted to Be*. Simon and Schuster, 2015.

CHAPTER TWO

SEX AND RELATIONSHIPS

Date Night at the Orgy Dome

LUBRICANTS

COCONUT OIL
You can buy it by the gallon!
https://store.nutiva.com/coconut-oil/

HYALO GYN
http://www.hyalogyn.com/

PROHYDRATE
http://vagisil.com/en-uk/products/prohydrate-internal-hydrating-gel/

ÜBERLUBE
My favorite silicone based
http://www.babeland.com/uberlube/d/4524#

VAGIFEM
https://www.vagifem.com/

MISCELLANEOUS

COSABELLA
For my go-to nightie.
https://www.cosabella.com

BURNING MAN
When you really need to spice things up
https://burningman.org/

SEX TOYS (A FEW FAVORITES)

CRAVE BULLET
http://www.lovecrave.com/vibrators/bullet/features

HITACHI MAGIC WAND
The original "personal massager"
https://hitachimagic.com/

CRAVE VESPER NECKLACE
Combination jewelry and vibrator! I wear my gold-toned one all the time and love the looks I get from certain other middle-aged women in the know.
http://store.lovecrave.com/vesper/

MIO BY JE JOUE
http://jejoue.com/which-toy/mio.html

RABBIT HABIT
A friend found one of these under her teenage daughter's bed and almost had a heart attack. But then she bought one for herself…
https://rabbitvibrators.net/

WE-VIBE
This one just never gets old.
http://we-vibe.com/

TO READ

Anonymous. *The Pearl*. Ballantine Books, 2006.

Bentley, Toni. *The Surrender*. Ecco, 2005.

Friday, Nancy. *My Secret Garden*. Quartet Books, 1998.

Jong, Erica. *Sugar in My Bowl: Real Women Write About Real Sex*. Ecco, 2011.

Kerner, Ian, PhD. *She Comes First: The Thinking Man's Guide to Pleasuring a Woman*. William Morrow, 2009.

Millet, Catherine. *The Sexual Life of Catherine M.* Grove Press, 2003.

Nagoski, Emily. *Come As You Are: The Surprising New Science That Will Transform Your Sex Life*. Simon and Schuster, 2015.

Nin, Anaïs. *Delta of Venus*. Harvest/HBJ, 1986.

Perel, Esther. *Mating in Captivity: Unlocking Erotic Intelligence*. Harper Paperbacks, 2007.

Reage, Pauline. *Story of O*. Ballantine Books, 2013.

Sprinkle, Annie. *An Explorer's Guide to Planet Orgasm*. Greenery Press, 2017.

Thomashauer, Regena. *Mama Gena's School of Womanly Arts*. Simon and Schuster, 2004.

Valenti, Jessica. *Sex Object: A Memoir*. Dey Street Books, 2017.

Venning, Rachel. *Moregasm: Babeland's Guide to Mind-Blowing Sex*. Morrow, 2010.

CHAPTER THREE

BODIES

Is Everything Sagging or Is It Just Me?

AMERICAN COLLEGE OF SPORTS MEDICINE
http://www.acsm.org/

AUTHORITY NUTRITION
Nutrition info
https://authoritynutrition.com/about/

FITBIT
https://www.fitbit.com/home

MAYO CLINIC
http://www.mayoclinic.org/

MEDITERRANEAN DIET
http://www.mayoclinic.org/healthy
-lifestyle/nutrition-and-healthy
-eating/in-depth/mediterranean
-diet/art-20047801

MENOPAUSE IN AN HOUR (DVD) BY DR. TARA ALLMAN
https://www.amazon.com/
Menopause-Hour-Dr-Tara-Allmen/
dp/B00746R3UI

METZL, DR. JORDAN
http://drjordanmetzl.com/

NATIONAL INSTITUTE ON ALCO-HOL AND ALCOHOL ABUSE
https://www.niaaa.nih.gov/

NIKE FUELBAND
http://www.nike.com/us/en_us/c/
nike-plus

QI GONG
https://www.youtube.com/
watch?v=3K-0JpiJu-o

SEVEN-MINUTE WORKOUT
So fun, so easy!
http://7-min.com/

WHOLE30
My go-to nutrition plan when I need to feel virtuous
https://whole30.
com/whole30-program-rules/

TO READ

Copeland, Misty. *Ballerina Body*. Grand Central, 2017.
Ephron, Nora. *I Feel Bad About My Neck*. Vintage, 2008.
Meltzer, Marisa. "Forget Body Positivity: How About Body Neutrality?" *New York*, March 1, 2017.

Northrup, Christiane. *Women's Bodies, Women's Wisdom.* Bantam, 2010.
Olds, Sharon. *Odes.* Knopf, 2016.
West, Lindy. *Shrill.* Hachette, 2017.

CHAPTER FOUR

PARENTING

A (Not Quite) Empty Nest

TO READ

Coburn, Karen, and Madge Lawrence Treeger. *Letting Go: A Parents' Guide to Understanding the College Years.* Harper Perennial, 2009.
Daum, Meghan. *Selfish, Shallow, and Self-Absorbed: Sixteen Writers on the Decision Not to Have Kids.* Picador, 2016.
Kindlon, Dan. *Raising Cain.* Ballantine, 2000.
Lamott, Anne. *Operating Instructions.* Anchor, 2005.
Orenstein, Peggy. *Girls & Sex: Navigating the Complicated New Landscape.* Harper Paperbacks, 2017.

CHAPTER FIVE

BEAUTY

Mirror, Mirror...?

AMERICAN SOCIETY OF PLASTIC SURGEONS
https://www.plasticsurgery.org

BRILLIANT DISTINCTIONS
For negligible discounts on Botox and fillers
https://www.brilliantdistinction sprogram.com/

DAY, DORIS, MD
http://www.myclearskin.com/

EYELASH EXTENSIONS
Where I go to get my lashes done
http://jjeyelashes.com/salons/

GOTTLIEB, MARTIN, DDS
http://www.godental365.com/

INGLETON, ROSEMARIE, MD
http://ingletonmd.com/

TINKLE RAZOR
So cheap and totally works!
http://tinkleyourface.com/

TWEEZERMAN
The only brand of tweezer worth buying, but you'll still need multiples.
https://www.tweezerman.com/

TO READ

Applewhite, Ashton. *This Chair Rocks: A Manifesto Against Ageism*. Networked Books, 2015.

Guiliano, Mireille. *French Women Don't Get Facelifts*. Grand Central Life & Style, 2013.

Kreamer, Anne. *Going Gray: How to Embrace Your Authentic Self with Grace and Style*. Little, Brown, and Company, 2009.

Wolf, Naomi. *The Beauty Myth*. Harper Perennial 2002.

CHAPTER SIX

EMOTIONS

Anxiety and Depression and Stress, Oh My!

BRACH, TARA
Meditation via laptop, for me
https://www.tarabrach.com/

BROWN, BRENÉ, PHD
If you aren't familiar with her work on vulnerability and shame, run to YouTube now.
http://brenebrown.com/

DYER, WAYNE, PHD
Fabulous books and podcasts
http://www.drwaynedyer.com/

HEADSPACE
https://www.headspace.com/

MAGIDS, DEBBIE, PHD
I couldn't love my therapist more.
https://www.drdebbie.com/

MENTAL HEALTH AMERICA
http://www.mentalhealthamerica.net/

THE MINDFULNESS APP
http://themindfulnessapp.com/

NATIONAL INSTITUTE OF MENTAL HEALTH
https://www.nimh.nih.gov/index.shtml

UNIVERSITY OF MICHIGAN DEPRESSION CENTER
http://www.depressioncenter.org/

PSYCHOLOGY TODAY
This website will help you locate therapists.
https://therapists.psychologytoday.com/rms

TO READ

Benjamin, Marina. *The Middlepause: On Turning Fifty*. Catapult, 2016.
de Beauvoir, Simone. *The Coming of Age*. W. W. Norton and Company, 1996.
Loh, Sandra Tsing. *The Madwoman in the Volvo: My Year of Raging Hormones*.
    W. W. Norton and Company, 2015.
Ruefle, Mary. *My Private Property*. Wave Books, 2016.
Segal, Lynne. *Out of Time: The Pleasures and Perils of Aging*. Verso, 2013.

CHAPTER SEVEN

HEALTH

Not What the Doctor Ordered

AMERICAN CANCER SOCIETY
https://www.cancer.org/

ARTHRITIS FOUNDATION
http://www.arthritis.org/

CENTERS FOR DISEASE CONTROL AND PREVENTION
https://www.cdc.gov/

CLEVELAND HEARING AND SPEECH CENTER
http://www.chsc.org/Main/Audiology.aspx

ELVIE
High-tech Kegel tool
https://www.elvie.com/

ICON PANTIES
Definitely the most stylish way to date to deal with incontinence.
https://www.iconundies.com/pages/incontinence-underwear-reviews

LIFT (SENSORY DEPRIVATION TANKS)
A novel way to meditate and provide self-care
http://www.liftfloats.com/

MEMORIAL SLOAN KETTERING CANCER CENTER
Great supplement section
https://www.mskcc.org/cancer-care/diagnosis-treatment/symptom-management/integrative-medicine/herbs

KEGEL CAMP APP
Hands down my fave way to remember to Kegel; I'm jealous I didn't think of this first.
https://itunes.apple.com/es/app/kegel-camp/id425190605?l=en&mt=8

NORTH AMERICAN MENOPAUSE SOCIETY (NAMS)
The leading nonprofit organization focused on women and aging; extensive resources
https://www.menopause.org

RESTORE YOUR CORE
https://laurenohayon.com/offerings/restore-your-core/

U.S. PREVENTIVE SERVICES TASK FORCE
https://www.uspreventiveservicestaskforce.org/

TO READ

Allmen, Tara. *Menopause Confidential*. HarperCollins, 2016.
Corio, Laura. *The Change Before the Change*. Penguin Random House, 2002.
Gurwitch, Annabelle. *I See You Made an Effort*. Penguin, 2014.
Huffington, Arianna. *The Sleep Revolution*. Penguin Random House, 2017.
Reiss, Uzzi. *Natural Hormone Balance for Women*. Atria, 2001.
Somers, Suzanne. *I'm Too Young for This*. Harmony, 2013.

CHAPTER EIGHT

WORK AND MONEY

But How Will I Pay for My Depends?

AARP
http://www.aarp.org/

ADLER, STEVEN
My estate planner, first met on Match.com!
http://www.sawlaw.com/

APRÈS
https://apresgroup.com/

CLAYMAN, AMANDA, FINANCIAL COACH
https://amandaclayman.com/

ENCORE
http://encore.org/

PATH FORWARD
http://pathforward.org/

RETIREMENT CALCULATOR
http://www.aarp.org/work/
retirement-planning/retirement
_calculator.html

SECOND SHIFT
https://www.thesecondshift.com/

**SOCIAL SECURITY BENEFITS
PLANNER**
https://www.ssa.gov/planners/
index.html

TO READ

Fels, Anna. *Necessary Dreams: Ambition in Women's Changing Lives*. Pantheon,
    2004.
Orman, Suze. *Women and Money: Owning the Power to Control Your Destiny*.
    Spiegel & Grau, 2007.
Robbins, Tony. *Money: Master the Game*. Simon & Schuster 2014.
Stewart, James. *Den of Thieves*. Simon & Schuster, 1991.

INDEX

(ABOUT THE AUTHOR)

NINA LOREZ COLLINS was born in New York City in 1969 and attended Barnard College. She had a long career in book publishing, first as a scout and then as an agent. She completed a master's in narrative medicine at Columbia University and became a certified life coach with IPEC. She has four children and lives in Brooklyn, where she is a trustee of the Brooklyn Public Library. Feel free to email her at nina@whatwouldvirginiawoolfdo.com and check out the website www.thewoolfer.com.